Shortness of Breath
A Guide to Better Living and Breathing

KENNETH M. MOSER, M.D.

ANDREW L. RIES, M.D.

DAWN E. SASSI-DAMBRON, R.N., B.S.N.

BIRGITTA K. ELLIS, P.T.

TRINA M. LIMBERG, B.S., R.R.T.

ROSEANN MYERS, R.N.

Pulmonary and Critical Care Division
University of California, San Diego,
School of Medicine
San Diego, California

FOURTH EDITION
with 103 illustrations by Steve Pileggi

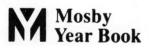 Mosby
Year Book

St. Louis   Baltimore   Boston   Chicago   London   Philadelphia   Sydney   Toronto

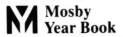

Mosby
Year Book

Dedicated to Publishing Excellence

Publisher: David Culverwell
Assistant Editorial: Cecilia F. Reilly
Editorial Project Manager: Jolynn Gower
Design Manager: Susan Lane
Production Editor: Kathy Lumpkin

FOURTH EDITION

Printed in the United States of America

Mosby-Year Book, Inc.
11830 Westline Industrial Drive
St. Louis, Missouri 63146

Library of Congress Cataloging-in-Publication Data

Shortness of breath: a guide to better living and breathing / Kenneth
    M. Moser . . . [et al.].—4th ed.
        p.   cm.
    Includes index.
    ISBN 0-8016-9055-2
    1. Lungs—Diseases, Obstructive—Popular works.   I. Moser,
Kenneth M., 1929-
RC776.03S53   1991   91-8956
616.2′4—dc20   CIP

Preface

Any book with multiple authors of different backgrounds must have an interesting story behind it, and this one does. The story begins more than 20 years ago, when we established one of the first Respiratory Intensive Care Units in the United States. Trying to save the lives of patients who had developed severe, life-threatening shortness of breath was a rewarding and exciting venture. Yet we soon recognized that many admissions to this Unit could have been avoided if the patient had been better educated about the causes of shortness of breath and how to deal with them. We decided that education was a vital and missing link in the health care system. Almost exclusively, patients appeared to be passive observers of their own health care. We became convinced that, with proper education, people could and should become active participants in their own health care.

But how could people acquire such education? Certainly not through medical textbooks, which were too technical and detailed. Nor through the standard media, which dealt only sporadically with the problem and rarely presented practical or scientifically sound information. Nor from most "health books," which usually presented a point of view rather than a body of facts. And not from busy physicians who, however well motivated, rarely had time to educate their patients.

So we concluded that such an educational effort could be provided most effectively by a respiratory care team that included individuals with a wide range of professional skills and knowledge: pulmonary physicians, pulmonary nursing specialists, respiratory therapists, chest physical therapists, cardiopulmonary technologists, psychiatrists, social workers, nutritionists, occupational therapists, and hospital administrators. This team would develop a course devoted to the education of patients with shortness of breath, emphasizing the most common cause of this symptom: chronic obstructive lung disease (COPD).

At that time, such ideas and approaches were controversial. Some felt that an educated patient might be more of a threat than a help to the health care system; others felt that people would not be interested in such self-education. Still others felt that such an effort would intrude on physician-patient relationships. Despite such reservations, the effort was undertaken.

The multidisciplinary team was developed, and together, they designed a course for people with shortness of breath. The first patients came and learned and benefited. The process was refined, changed, and repeated, and a gratifying dividend appeared. As the years and courses passed, many physicians and allied health professionals visited our program to learn the course elements and begin similar efforts at their offices, clinics, and hospitals.

But an increasing source of frustration to us was that our educational efforts were still reaching a relatively small audience. Our program was consistently "backlogged," so that we could reach only a modest percentage of the interested individuals in our immediate geographic area, and extension of our program to other areas was not feasible.

This book was a logical means for extending our educational efforts to the larger audience that we could never personally reach. So, that is the story behind the first edition of this book, which appeared in 1975. Five years later, in 1980, the second edition was published and, in 1983, the third, each incorporating certain new concepts and treatments that had developed in the interim. The quick pace of medical advancement has now catalyzed this fourth edition, and we have added information of interest to individuals with lung diseases other than COPD. Indeed, such broadening of the audience fits with an exciting new development: the potential of heart-lung and lung transplantation for many patients with shortness of breath at our institution and others. Participation in a rehabilitation program is a key element in the preparation of such patients for surgery—and in their postoperative maintenance.

Over the years, this book—like all aspects of medical care—has changed. One thing, however, has not changed; indeed, it has become stronger. That is our belief that patients with shortness of breath can become active members of the treatment team, accepting (and enjoying) the fact that they can and must play a central role in their own care. That is still the theme of this book. In fact, since 1975, that theme has become a national one in the area of health care: the individual's active participation in the goal of maintaining and improving his or her health.

We hope that all of our colleagues in respiratory care will continue to find this book useful and that patients with shortness of breath will learn from its pages how to live better and more functional lives.

Of course, despite the multiple authorship, many others have contributed directly or indirectly to this book. We owe special debts of gratitude to Steve Pileggi, whose illustrations have contributed so much to our programs and this book; Drs. Allen Abrams and Sharon Grodner, whose devotion to the mental health of our patients has helped them (and us) live better lives; Kelly L. Mosier, our Dietician, who has taught us all much about nutrition; Drs. Raffi I. Simonian and Charles L. James, for sharing their expertise in pharmacology; Carol Archibald, R.N., M.S.N., Donna Whelan, R.R.T., Patsy Hansen, R.N., M.S.N., Jamie Sheldon, P.T., and Lela Prewitt, whose efforts have helped shape and sustain our program and this volume; Dr. Jack Clausen, Kathy Fonzi, Donna Elliott and the entire technical crew in the UCSD Pulmonary Physiology Laboratory; a succession of pulmonary trainees and students at UCSD who have been our teachers as well as our students; Joyce Sly and Carol Howard, who have borne the administrative burden of translating our ideas into readable copy; and finally, our patients, who have continued to return more to us than we have given them.

Kenneth M. Moser, M.D.

Note to the Reader

A number of medications, exercises, and other forms of medical treatment are reviewed in this book. While the descriptions are as accurate as possible, they should not be taken as direct instruction or recommendation for any individual patient. The contents of this book are informational only. Any specific medication or exercise should be prescribed by a physician and initiated under appropriate medical guidance.

Contents

1

What's Shortness of Breath All About?

Most of us take breathing for granted. Like the beating of the heart, breathing just happens automatically. When we exercise, we know our breathing quickens and deepens, just as our pulse rate increases. But again, we don't have to think about these things. We decide what we want to do and somehow the lungs (and heart) follow along.

The fancy medical word for feeling short of breath is *dyspnea* (pronounced disp-nee-ah). Dyspnea is a difficult symptom for people to deal with because it is a feeling, a sensation. Only the individual knows that he or she is experiencing shortness of breath. The physician also has trouble evaluating dyspnea. Often it cannot be detected on physical examination. There is no specific test for it. Therefore the individual must report dyspnea to the physician. In many ways, dyspnea is like pain—a symptom that only the patient feels and can describe. Pain and dyspnea are invisible to others.

Like pain, shortness of breath is experienced differently by different people. Some individuals have a very high threshold for pain, some a very low one. It is the same with dyspnea. Some people who appear to others to

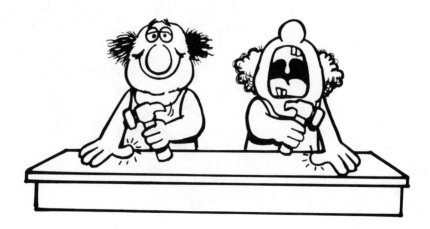

be short of breath do not themselves feel dyspneic. Other individuals feel quite short of breath when they appear to be breathing normally. Just why this is cannot be fully explained. There are probably multiple reasons.

When Is Shortness of Breath Abnormal?

Shortness of breath is a tricky symptom. To compound the problem, everyone feels short of breath sometimes. Even the well-conditioned athlete with excellent lung and heart function experiences dyspnea. So how do you know when shortness of breath is abnormal? When is it a possible signal of disease? When should you have it checked out by a doctor?

Here are some simple tests to apply:

(1) Are you more short of breath doing certain things than are other people your own age? It is obviously not abnormal when a 60-year-old man or woman feels short of breath while playing tennis with a 20-year-old son or daughter. It is not abnormal to feel short of breath if you lead a quite sedentary life and suddenly try to run a mile. But it is abnormal if you feel short of breath walking up an incline or up stairs when people of your own age (co-workers, friends, or spouse) do not. Comparison with peers is a key test.

(2) Are you short of breath doing things that a few months or a year ago you could do easily without this feeling? Do you now avoid the stairs at work or home because of shortness of breath? In asking these questions,

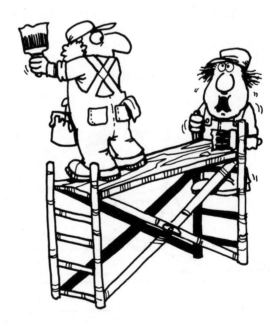

you are comparing you with yourself. The questions should be answered honestly. Denying such changes won't make them go away.

(3) Have you experienced a *sudden* change? Suddenly feeling short of breath while resting or being active is almost always abnormal. A rapid change like this merits prompt medical attention.

Asking these questions usually distinguishes normal from abnormal shortness of breath. However, sometimes an individual either does not ask these questions or denies that the answers are "yes." In such situations, other people may have to call the problem to your attention. They notice that you are breathing hard during a walk at a pace that is leisurely for them. Spouses are often the first to notice such things. If friends or a spouse poses these questions to you, take them seriously rather than explaining them away (which is easy to do). You may have a "high threshold" for dyspnea, but if you are changing your behavior to avoid shortness of breath, others may be more aware of it than you are. Or maybe you are aware, but don't want to admit it as long as you believe that no one else notices.

Check It Out

However shortness of breath is called to your attention, it is better to take it seriously than to push it out of your mind. Taking it seriously means seeing a physician. The doctor can then check out whether the shortness of breath is normal or abnormal for you. As with most symptoms, delay in finding out about dyspnea is not wise. If there is something wrong, valuable time may be lost, time during which the chance for effective treatment may pass. If there is *not* something wrong, if you or others around you just have a "low threshold," then finding that out will relieve your mind—and theirs. So "when in doubt, check it out."

What Causes Shortness of Breath?

If shortness of breath is a signal of disease, what are the possible problems involved? Well, there are a lot of possibilities—just as there are a lot of causes of pain. For example, anemia can make people short of breath, and anemia has multiple causes. Being overweight can cause dyspnea, as can certain glandular problems, such as an overactive or underactive thyroid gland. Heart diseases of various types are a frequent cause of shortness of breath—without chest pains or any other symptoms. But the most common reason for shortness of breath is lung disease.

All of the causes of shortness of breath can usually be sorted out by having a physician take a careful history, perform a complete physical examination, and obtain certain simple laboratory tests: a blood count, a chest x-ray examination, and an electrocardiogram. Sometimes more extensive

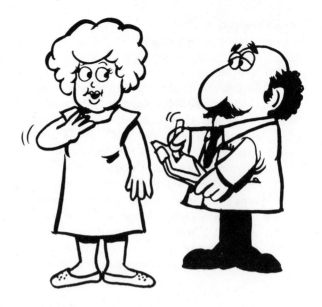

tests are needed to find out whether anything is really wrong and, if so, what it is. But the doctor also should take your symptom seriously, not dismiss it with a statement that "you are getting older" or are "out of shape." The history and physical examination should be carefully done, and at least the three tests mentioned should be performed.

What Kinds of Lung Disease Are There?

If this sequence has been followed, and if the reason for your shortness of breath turns out to be the most common one—lung disease—you will want to know what kinds of lung diseases there are and what needs to be done to find out which kind you have.

There are many diseases that can affect the lungs and lead to shortness of breath. Most of them, particularly the ones with long and complex names, are rare. But despite the many possibilities, lung diseases can be grouped into three main categories: restrictive diseases that reduce the volume of the lungs, diseases that injure and/or block the blood vessels of the lungs, and obstructive diseases that make it difficult to expel air from the lungs (slow down exhalation).

The restrictive diseases cause shortness of breath by either scarring the lungs or filling their air spaces. Usually these diseases are slow and progressive—and so is the shortness of breath they produce. Sometimes the cause for this chronic irritation and scarring of the lungs is known: exposure to asbestos, beryllium, or other injurious fumes or particles, or allergic reaction to certain inhaled materials such as cotton dust or pigeon droppings.

Such inhalation exposure most often occurs at work but may occur at home. Many of the restrictive diseases are of unknown cause. These are grouped under the term *idiopathic*—a terrific medical term that means "of unknown cause." A common form of restrictive lung disease is "idiopathic interstitial pneumonitis." This means that the patient has an inflammation of the lung (pneumonitis) that involves the connective tissue of the lung (interstitium) and is of unknown cause. But whether the cause is known or unknown, a diagnosis can be made and a treatment program started. Because scarring may occur, and scars cannot be reversed, an early diagnosis is important—before the scarring and other lung injuries do become severe and irreversible.

Diseases of the lung blood vessels are less common. They develop because of injury to the small lung blood vessels or because blood clots (called emboli) block off the larger pulmonary vessels. Shortness of breath—sometimes developing suddenly, sometimes gradually—is usually the only symptom. Often these diseases go undiagnosed for long periods because patients "adapt" to their breathing limitations and therefore feel nothing is wrong. But, again, this is a mistake because early diagnosis and treatment are vital.

By far the most common lung diseases are of the obstructive type. That is why the rest of this book is devoted almost exclusively to them. Except for asthma, these diseases tend to cause shortness of breath mostly in people beyond age 40—and this dyspnea is all too often attributed to "age" or "being out of shape." Therefore diagnosis is often long delayed because the individual does not seek medical attention.

The Central Points

This brief summary of the causes of shortness of breath is far from comprehensive. Whole books can be written (and have been!) about any one of them. The central points are these:

- Shortness of breath may be a signal of disease.
- To determine whether it *is* such a signal requires evaluation by a doctor.
- A good history, physical examination, and simple laboratory tests can usually tell you and the doctor whether disease is present, and if so, what it is.
- Early diagnosis of all the diseases—including those of the lung—is important because delay in diagnosis means delay in treatment.
- Delay in treatment may lead to irreversible changes in the lungs (and, in some instances, in the heart as well).
- Of the lung diseases that cause shortness of breath, the "obstructive" ones are the most common.

This manual is primarily for individuals with obstructive lung disease. Some parts also apply to people with other kinds of lung diseases. If you have a lung disease other than asthma, chronic bronchitis, or emphysema, your physician can tell you which parts of the book apply to you and which do not. Don't make a self-diagnosis. Proper understanding of your problem and its treatment begins with establishing a firm diagnosis. That is the physician's job. Don't try to do it for him or her.

2

The Lungs: How They Are Put Together and How They Work

To understand your disease, you should know how normal lungs are built and how they work. Then it is easier to recognize what has happened to your lungs, why you get certain symptoms, and what you and your doctor can do to improve these symptoms. Some new vocabulary is involved. If you learn these new words, you will be able to talk with your doctor more easily and not be confused by things he says or articles you may read about lung disease.

How the Body's Engine Runs

The human body was designed to run on oxygen as its "energy" source, just as automobile engines run on gasoline or diesel fuel and power plants run on coal, oil, or other fuels. And, just as with other fuels, when the body "burns" oxygen for energy, waste products result: the two major waste products are water and carbon dioxide.

Therefore all of the body's functions depend on delivery of a steady supply of oxygen. Unfortunately, the body cannot store much oxygen. If delivery stops, the body, "runs out of gas (oxygen)" within about 5 minutes. So the supply must be continuous, unlike the supply of food or water.

Furthermore, the waste products must be excreted promptly. Getting rid of water presents no problems. If the body retains water, it can still function and, sooner or later, excrete (get rid of) it through the kidneys as urine or through the sweat glands. But if carbon dioxide builds up in the body, it creates acids in the blood. An excess of such acids can impair the function of important organs such as the brain and heart. And a build-up of carbon dioxide can produce symptoms such as headaches, drowsiness, and fatigue.

The lungs are designed to solve the twin problems of continuous oxygen delivery and carbon dioxide removal. They are the only route by which oxygen can be delivered to the body. Acids and carbon dioxide can be excreted by the kidneys, but the lungs get rid of carbon dioxide (and prevent acidity) much more quickly and efficiently than do the kidneys.

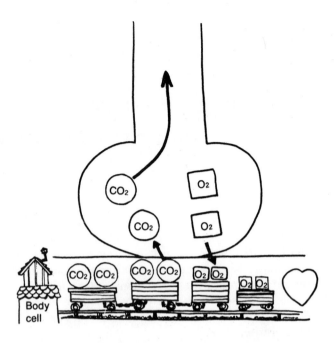

To carry out these two vital functions, the lungs need to have a practical way to bring fresh air (inspired air) into contact with the blood in a safe manner so that the blood can pick up oxygen and get rid of excess carbon dioxide. Then the air must be efficiently expelled (expired) into the environment and the blood pumped to the rest of the body.

How the Lungs Are Designed

Step one: Getting air in and out

This function is carried out by a system of branching air tubes (bronchial tubes) to bring air in and out of the lungs, and a system of blood tubes (pulmonary arteries) to bring blood to the lungs. The system of air tubes is called the *bronchial tree,* an appropriate name because it looks like an upside-down tree. It begins with a single, large tube (like the tree "trunk") called the *windpipe,* or *trachea,* which you can feel with your fingers in your neck. The trachea extends from the back of the mouth to the inside of the chest (or *thorax*). There, the trachea divides into two major branches (one to the right lung and one to the left lung). Next, each of these main stem bronchi branches many times into smaller and smaller bronchial tubes, just as a tree branches. When the branches become very small (so small that they can be seen only with a microscope), they are given a new name: *bronchioles.*

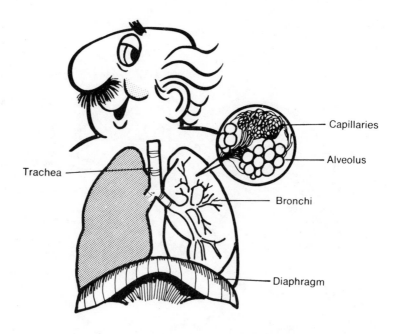

The larger bronchial tubes have cartilage in their walls. Cartilage is a rigid but flexible material—flexible enough to change shape as we breathe but rigid enough to prevent the larger bronchial tubes from collapsing. The smaller bronchial tubes have no cartilage in their walls; they are surrounded by a circle of muscle. If this muscle contracts, the tubes can be greatly narrowed. All bronchial tubes are lined by a delicate layer of cells (the *mucous membrane*). Some of the cells in this membrane produce a sticky fluid called *mucus*, which coats the mucous membrane. Some of the cells also have hairlike structures on them *(cilia)*, which beat rhythmically. The mucus lies on top of these cilia—a fact we shall talk more about later on.

The bronchioles also branch and finally end in a cluster of little balloon-like structures called the *air sacs*, or *alveoli*. There are about 300 million of these alveoli in the lungs. Thus one trachea leads to 300 million alveoli; clearly, that involves a lot of branching! The alveoli have extremely thin walls. They also contain "elastic" tissue in their walls, making them behave much like tiny rubber balloons.

Step two: Getting blood in and out

The system of blood tubes is similar in structure. It begins with one large tube *(main pulmonary artery)* that comes out of the right side of the heart *(right ventricle)*. The main artery then splits into a right and left branch,

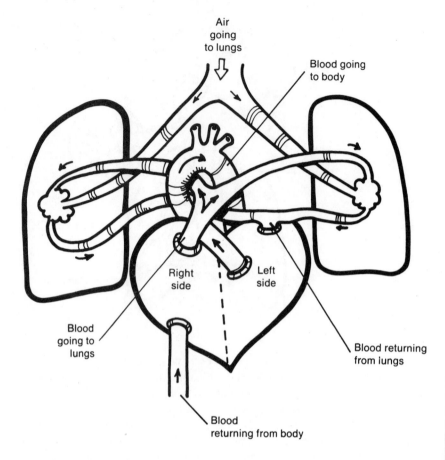

Air
going
to lungs

Blood going
to body

Blood going to
lungs

Right
side

Left
side

Blood returning
from lungs

Blood
returning from body

one supplying each lung. Then each of these branches, like those in the bronchial system, divides many times into smaller and smaller pulmonary arteries. The smallest branches of this system also get a new name: *arterioles*. The arterioles run along the walls of the bronchioles. Finally, the arterioles reach the alveoli; there they divide again into tiny vessels called *capillaries*. The capillaries are in the walls of the alveoli. Therefore the blood in the capillaries is separated from the air in the alveoli only by the extremely thin, elastic walls of the alveoli. This is why it is normally so easy for oxygen to get into, and carbon dioxide to get out of, the blood. There are about 1 billion capillaries, more than three to each air sac.

Once the blood has passed through the capillaries (and taken up new oxygen and disposed of excess carbon dioxide), it goes to the left side of the heart *(left atrium* and *ventricle)*. The left ventricle now pumps this "fresh" blood to the organs of the body through the arteries. Therefore the arteries contain blood that has just come from the lungs. If the lungs are working properly, this blood contains a normal amount of oxygen and carbon dioxide; if they are not, the amount of oxygen and carbon dioxide may be abnormal—the oxygen decreased and the carbon dioxide increased. That is why blood is often taken from arteries and analyzed; these *arterial blood gas values* tell your doctor whether your lungs are doing their job.

There is often confusion in peoples' minds about the "right side" and the "left side" of the heart. Although both sides are in one package (the heart) in your chest, you now know that the right heart pumps blood to the lungs; the left side receives this "fresh" blood and pumps it to the rest of the body. Therefore the right heart can be directly affected by lung diseases. The left heart cannot. The blood in your arm or leg *veins* is returning to the right heart to be pumped to the lungs. The veins are bluish and do not pulsate. Your arm or leg *arteries* contain blood that has just come from the lungs and is on its way to your organs (for instance, the brain, kidney, and muscles). The arteries usually cannot be seen except as pulsations, but these pulsations are easily felt.

How the "Respiratory Pump" Works

There are a few more things you should know about how the lungs work. For example, what makes air go into *(inspiration)* and out of *(expiration)* the lungs? The elastic lungs are contained within an airtight box called the chest, or thorax. The chest is sealed at its lower end by the *diaphragm*, a thin muscle that separates the chest from the abdomen ("stomach cavity"). The diaphragm moves up and down like a piston. When it moves down (inspiration), the airtight thorax expands and a slight vacuum (negative pressure) is created. Air from the outside is therefore sucked into the lungs to overcome this vacuum. The elastic alveoli are stretched, like expanding balloons; then the diaphragm relaxes and moves upward. The thorax becomes smaller, as do the elastic alveoli, which—again acting like balloons—expel the air from the lungs.

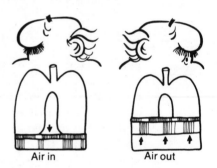

Air in   Air out

For this system to work, it must be airtight so that a vacuum can be created during respiration. To assure this airtightness, the inner side of the chest wall and the outer side of the lungs are covered by a thin membrane (sheet of cells) called the *pleura*, which is moistened by a tiny amount of fluid so that the lungs slide smoothly as the thorax (chest wall) expands and contracts.

Naturally, we are usually not aware of these things. Breathing normally goes on without our thinking about it, but as you know or will learn here, that is not the case if the lungs become abnormal. When the lungs become abnormal, muscles other than the diaphragm may be used to make the thorax larger and smaller. These are the intercostal muscles (which are between the ribs) and several muscles in the neck called *accessory muscles*. Usually, these muscles have little work to do during breathing; but in lung disease, they may have to do a great deal of work in breathing.

What "Controls" Breathing?

There is another thing that most of us do not think about when we breathe. How do we know how *much* to breathe? What controls *how deep* and *how fast* we breathe? Actually, we have a complicated "control" system built into the body that works a lot like a thermostat for regulating a central heating and cooling system. The usual thermostat registers temperature and turns the heater or air conditioner on or off to keep the temperature where you want it. The "breathing thermostat" senses the oxygen and carbon dioxide in the blood. It turns the breathing apparatus on and off (or makes it go faster or slower) to keep oxygen and carbon dioxide in the blood at proper levels. If the oxygen level in the blood falls, or if the carbon dioxide rises, this "thermostat" makes you breathe harder (quicker and deeper). That is why, for example, when people go to a high altitude where the amount of oxygen in the air is less, they breath faster and deeper.

How the Lungs Are Protected

Finally, there are some things you should know about how the lungs protect themselves against impurities and other changes in the air we breathe. As you know, the air around us can be hot or cold or wet or dry, and it can contain various irritating gases and particles. The lungs are delicate and work best when the air in them is *moist*, is at *body temperature* (37° C [98.6° F]), and is free of particles or irritating gases. Nature has designed several "protective" systems so that the lungs receive such air. The first of these systems is the *upper air passages*—the nose, the mouth, and the back of the mouth (oropharynx) where air entering the mouth or nose comes together. Above and around the nose and mouth are some "spaces" built into the skull called *sinuses*. These upper air passages and sinuses have two jobs: (1) to regulate the temperature and wetness of the air you breathe in and (2) to remove irritating particles and gases from this air. If the system works, air entering your windpipe will be at just the right temperature and wetness and will be free of impurities. Thus the upper air passages can warm or cool inhaled air and can add or remove water from it; furthermore, irritant gases or particles are "trapped" in the mucus that coats these passages and are then removed by cough, sneeze, expectoration, or nose blowing.

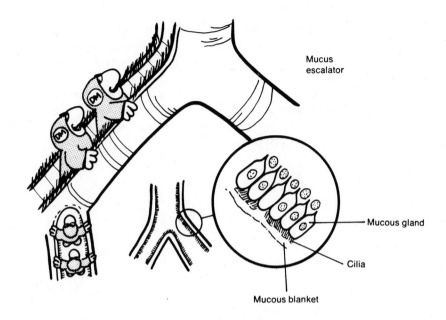

Mucus escalator

Mucous gland

Cilia

Mucous blanket

If the upper air passages fail or are unable to do these things properly, air enters the lungs in less than perfect condition. The lungs themselves have several protective systems that then swing into action. The mucous membranes of the air tubes also are equipped to warm or cool air and to adjust its wetness. Particles or irritants also are "trapped" in the mucus that coats the bronchial tubes. After they are trapped, they can be coughed out or, more commonly, removed by a "mucus escalator" built into the lungs. There is an "escalator" in the bronchial tree that consists of the mucous layer; this mucous layer is propelled from the small tubes to the windpipe by the *cilia* that beat toward the windpipe. The mucus is then either swallowed (without our being aware of it) or coughed out.

Of course, *cough* is another protection. Cough is produced by irritation of the bronchial tubes. This expels mucus much more rapidly than the "escalator." Cough also may alert us to the fact that we are inhaling irritating things and tell us to move away from them (if possible). Another "protection" is bronchial spasm. With severe irritation, the bronchial muscles contract, even in normal people. This is the body's way of trying to protect us from inhaling irritants (by clamping down the small bronchial tubes). The sensation is an unpleasant one; but again, it may alert us to an irritant exposure from which we should escape.

Finally, some irritating gases or particles may defy these elaborate protective systems and get to the air sacs. Even then, another defense system exists—a special kind of white blood cell called *macrophages*. These cells wander through the air sacs searching for debris—viruses, bacteria, and particles that were inhaled. They engulf (suck up) such things, carry them off, and digest them. These cells cannot carry away all inhaled irritants. Some irritants stay in the lungs and may cause future scarring or other problems.

This, then, is the way the normal lungs work and how they are constructed. Knowing about these things should help you to understand how to take care of your lungs and how, when they are injured or abnormal, to help them to work better.

3

COPD—What Does That Mean?

As has already been indicated, there are many lung diseases. The most common type of lung disease is obstructive lung disease. This is often referred to as *COPD*, which stands for Chronic Obstructive Pulmonary Disease. This term refers to a group of diseases that all share one common feature: difficulty in expelling air from the lungs. This is called *expiratory obstruction*.

There are three disease processes that are lumped together under the label of COPD: chronic bronchitis, emphysema, and asthma. Although each of these diseases develops differently, all cause expiratory obstruction. For patients, distinction among these three disorders is not critical because most individuals with COPD have some combination, and many of the symptoms and treatments are the same. (However, for research purposes, distinction among the COPDs remains of importance.)

Chronic Bronchitis

The problem in chronic bronchitis results from chronic inflammation and swelling of the cells lining the inside of the bronchi (air tubes). When inflamed, these cells produce excess quantities of mucus. The swelling of these cells narrows the air tubes, making breathing more difficult. The excess mucus narrows the tubes further and even blocks some completely. The irritation and excess mucus often cause chronic cough, which is an attempt to expectorate the mucus. The lungs also become more easily infected because of these abnormalities. With repeated infections, lung damage may occur. Airways may become permanently dilated (bronchiectasis). Alveoli may become scarred (fibrosis). The narrowing of the bronchial tubes makes it more difficult for air to move in and out of them. If some tubes become blocked with mucus, the air sacs they supply cannot receive oxygen or get rid of carbon dioxide; they may, at least temporarily, collapse.

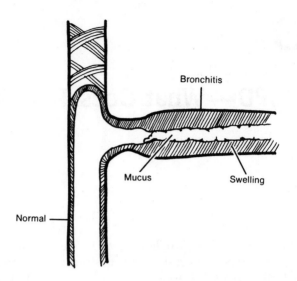

Emphysema

Emphysema is a disease in which the walls of the alveoli (air sacs) fracture (break). As these walls rupture, one large air sac replaces two, four, or many more small ones. The result is that the number of air sacs (alveoli) is reduced and many of those that remain are enlarged. One large sac is less elastic than the many tiny sacs were. Thus the patient with emphysema has lungs of *reduced elasticity*. To visualize the problems this causes, think of how a balloon works. You must blow (work) to fill it. But when you stop blowing, the balloon recoils (deflates) without your doing anything. The

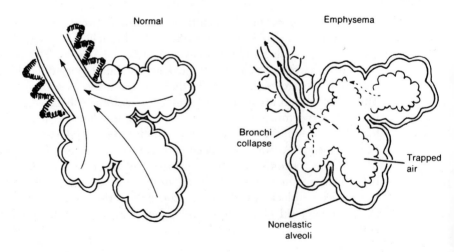

balloon's own elasticity causes it to expel the air. This is how normal alveoli work. You work (inspire) to inflate them with air. But when you relax, the lungs recoil (deflate) without effort on your part. Expiration (blowing air out of the lungs) is, therefore, a passive event. It just happens.

In emphysema the lungs and alveoli behave more like a paper bag. When you blow air into a paper bag, then stop blowing, what happens? Nothing. The bag stays full of air because it is nonelastic; it does not recoil. To empty the air from a paper bag, you must squeeze it out—and you must expend effort to push the air out. People with emphysema must do the same thing: expend energy during expiration to squeeze air out of the lungs.

Furthermore, this loss of lung elasticity affects the smaller bronchial tubes. To push air out of these less elastic lungs, a higher pressure must be developed inside the chest. This higher pressure tends to collapse the smaller bronchial tubes, making it even harder to empty air from the alveoli. Worsened expiratory obstruction results as the "neck of the balloon" (the bronchial tube) becomes narrowed. This tendency of the bronchial tubes to collapse also occurs with cough and makes it more difficult for the individual to cough up mucus. This collection of mucus, in turn, makes the lungs more susceptible to infection.

Asthma

The problem in asthma is that some irritant makes the muscles of the bronchial tubes go into spasm. This spasm narrows the bronchial tubes. Often this same irritant causes the lining cells of the bronchial tubes to swell and increase their production of mucus (secretions). These changes further narrow and clog up the bronchial tubes. When these things happen, the individual notices sudden shortness of breath and sometimes wheezing and cough.

There are several irritants that produce asthma. One is an *allergen*—that is, some material to which the patient is allergic. An allergy can show

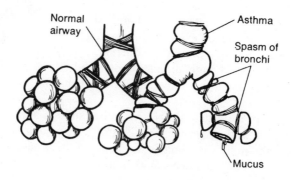

up as a rash, as an upset stomach, or as bronchial spasm (asthma). Infection is another source of irritation; cold air, smog, and cigarette smoke are others.

Many individuals with asthma have bronchial muscles that are more irritable than normal. Therefore small amounts of inhaled irritants can cause bronchial spasm in them but not in other people. This "hyperirritability" of the bronchial tubes may run in families (that is, it may be inherited).

COPD—How Do You Get It?

The causes of chronic obstructive lung disease have not been definitely determined. It is likely that the causes of emphysema, chronic bronchitis, and asthma are quite different. However, some features are common to each. For example, heredity seems to play a role in the tendency to develop each disorder.

Air pollution, exposure to occupational dust and fumes, and lung infections make all forms of COPD worse. Allergy plays a role in some people with asthma but not in emphysema or bronchitis. Most of these things cannot be controlled by the affected person. But one factor is under the individual's control: cigarette smoking. Emphysema and chronic bronchitis rarely develop in nonsmokers; asthma is worsened by cigarette smoking.

COPD—What Are the Symptoms?

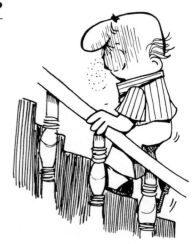

Usually the first thing a person with emphysema notices is shortness of breath on exertion (as when climbing stairs or walking quickly). As noted in Chapter 1, this symptom often is disregarded, and the individual feels it just means he or she is "out of shape" or "getting older." The first symptoms of chronic bronchitis are cough and mucus production. These symptoms are like a "chest cold" that hangs on week after week. Later, shortness of breath on exertion develops. The cough, mucus (sputum) production, and shortness of breath all may become suddenly worse if the individual develops the "flu" or some other type of lung infection.

. Asthma usually starts with rather sudden attacks of cough, shortness of breath, and wheezing. These attacks may come and go at first. Later on, cough, mild wheezing, and shortness of breath may be present all the time. The attacks may come on more frequently at certain times of the year (particularly spring or fall) after exposure to known allergens or irritants, only during exercise, or with the onset of a "cold." However, wheezing attacks also may appear without an obvious cause.

COPD—How Do You Know You Have It?

The diagnosis of COPD involves many factors. The first step is for you to consult your doctor if you have any of the symptoms of COPD. The most common symptom is shortness of breath, particularly on exertion (walking up steps, carry packages, hurrying during level walking). People often first notice that they "can't keep up with" their spouses or friends. A chronic cough or wheezing may be 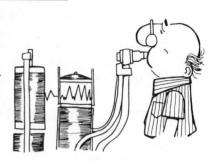 other symptoms. However, problems *other than COPD* can cause similar symptoms. Trouble breathing, like pain in the chest, can mean many different things.

Your doctor will carry out a physical examination and other tests, such as pulmonary function tests, to determine whether you have COPD or some other problems. The pulmonary function tests usually include breath-

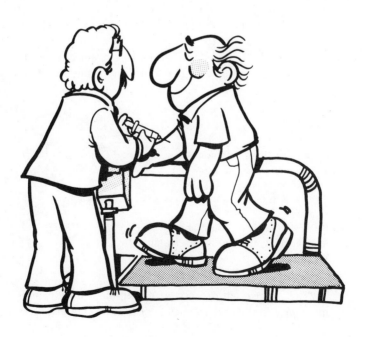

ing into one or more machines that measure how well your lungs are working. Also, a small blood sample may be taken from an artery while you rest and during exercise to determine how well the lungs are delivering oxygen to the blood and removing carbon dioxide from it. A chest x-ray examination is made to help this evaluation, but it cannot alone be used to diagnose COPD or other causes of lung symptoms. Using this evaluation as a basis, your doctor can then develop a proper treatment plan designed for you. The same tests can separate COPD from the other diseases that cause shortness of breath. So, no matter which kind of lung disease you have, the chest x-ray examination and pulmonary function tests provide valuable information.

COPD—What Can Be Done About It?

The most important factor in your treatment is the relationship you have with your doctor. You must be willing to be frank and honest, and your doctor must be the same with you. Some parts of your treatments will be the doctor's responsibility, such as prescribing drugs, treatments, tests, and diets. A big responsibility is yours. You must take the medicines as ordered, do your treatments at home, practice proper breathing, eat correctly, and most important of all, quit smoking if you haven't already. The treatment of COPD is a cooperative venture. Each person's disease is different.

Only your doctor knows which treatments and therapies are right for you. But only you know how you feel and how you respond to various treatments. Work with your doctor; ask questions. The more you know about your disease, the better off you are. The more your doctor knows about you, the better the treatment program that can be planned for you.

The treatment of COPD may include some or all of the following:

Medications
Adequate diet
Good hydration (fluid intake)
Use of respiratory therapy
Proper breathing techniques
Maintenance of muscle tone
Graded physical activity
Bronchial drainage to remove excess
  mucus
Prevention and treatment of infections
Avoidance of allergens and/or irritants
Weight control
Use of supplemental oxygen in some cases

The precise nature of your condition will determine the type of treatment prescribed. Sometimes very limited medication is all that is needed.

Sometimes rather extensive treatment is required. The aims of treatment are to reverse the reversible, to preserve the function you have, to prevent complications, and to teach you how to use the function you have more efficiently. These aims can be achieved whether your problem is mild or severe.

COPD—What is Your Responsibility?

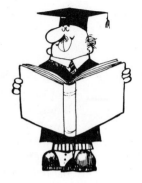

Now that you have an understanding of what COPD means and the goals of treatment, it's time to add the most important ingredient—*you*. With enthusiasm, perseverance, and knowledge, you can play a big role in controlling your disease and alleviating some of your symptoms. The remainder of this manual is devoted to all aspects of treatment. After your doctor has outlined the various therapies you are to use, consult your manual for guidance and review.

4

Understanding Your Medications

Many people with lung disease are given medications to take. It is important to know why the medications are being prescribed, exactly how to take them, and what positive or negative reactions to them may occur. People are often afraid to take certain medications—and secretly don't take them. That is not in their best interest. A lot of incorrect information is dispensed by friends, relatives, and people without medical training. Discuss each medicine with your doctor or pharmacist, both of whom will give you good information about all medications.

A number of different medications are used to treat persons with the various types of COPD. Each medicine is designed to do a specific job to help the lungs function more effectively. Your doctor will determine which medications you need on the basis of your history, physical examination, breathing tests, and other laboratory studies.

All medicines are chemicals. They may come from plant sources or from animals. Some drugs are made entirely by man—these are "synthesized" drugs. Medicines are used for their beneficial effects, but they may also cause side effects: a medicine taken by mouth must enter the stomach and then the blood in order to reach the lungs. Not only can medicines upset the stomach, but they also pass through many other organs while on their way to the lungs and may exert other effects, called *side effects*. Usually, these effects are well tolerated and may disappear with time. You should be familiar with what your medicine is supposed to do and with its side effects.

Another important fact to remember is that each medicine has two names: a generic (chemical) name and a brand (company) name. The generic name is always the same for each drug, no matter which company manufactures it. The brand name for a drug is the property of the company that markets that drug. In some states it is possible for your pharmacist to substitute a less expensive generic brand drug for the more expensive branded product. Sometimes the practice may cause you some confusion and you may think you have received the incorrect prescription. If there are any questions because the pills look different to you, consult with your pharmacist. Besides providing you with medicines, many pharmacies provide other helpful services. For example, many pharmacists maintain a complete record of all prescriptions you have received from any physician, dentist, or podiatrist. This "patient profile" can then be reviewed periodically by the pharmacist for drug interactions—a situation that occurs when two or more drugs taken at the same time work against each other. Ask your pharmacist or physician to explain this in more detail.

After each category of medication that follows, list, with the help of your physician or nurse, the names of the medications you take. They will be able to discuss the specific drugs with you. Include in your list the dose and time schedule for each drug. Then, carry this list with you at all times. Review and update it with your doctor at each visit.

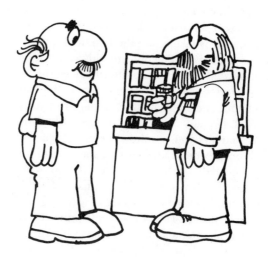

Bronchodilators

Bronchodilators relax the muscles of the breathing tubes, thereby making them wider and allowing air to get in and out more easily. Bronchodilators can be taken as pills, liquids, or aerosol sprays (see Chapter 5). The most common of these drugs are theophylline (a xanthine drug) and adrenergic drugs (adrenaline-like drugs). There are many different preparations of these types of drugs. Newer medications tend to be safer, easier to use, and more effective. The xanthine drugs may cause an upset stomach and heartburn. Others of these drugs, depending on how they are taken (pill or spray) and on how much you use, can increase your heart rate, make you feel jittery or nervous, or cause muscle tremors. Anticholinergic drugs (atropine-like drugs) are a new class of bronchodilator medicines currently used; in inhaled form, they may be better tolerated by you than other bronchodilators.

Steroids

Steroid drugs are all "relatives" of the hormone *cortisol*, which is normally produced by your body. These corticosteroids help to dilate the bronchial tubes and decrease swelling of the bronchial tube lining; they also help to decrease lung inflammation. Steroids have many potential side effects. They may make you feel very energetic and give you a (false) sense of well-being. Other common side effects include weight gain, redistribution of fat, and easy bruising. The side effects depend on the dose of the drug taken, how it is taken, and the length of time the therapy is continued. You must never discontinue oral steroids yourself or alter the dose without your physician's advice. People often hear stories about the side effects of steroids—stories that worry them. Remember that side effects are related to the amount and the schedule of *any* drug you take. Steroids are no different. And, like any drug, they are prescribed only when you need them and in the amounts you require. For many years, steroids could be taken only by pill or injection. Now certain special steroids have been developed that can be inhaled as an aerosol, directly into the lungs. They are absorbed very slowly and poorly into the blood. Therefore they have beneficial effects on the lungs while causing very few side effects. For people who need only small doses of steroids, these inhalations may replace oral steroids. However, all steroids must be taken on a regular schedule because they do not give immediate effects. Because they *prevent* bronchospasm, they are not to be used as you "need" them; instead, they should be taken *regularly* to prevent symptoms. Remember, these are potent medicines and must be taken only under the direction of your physician.

Cromolyn Sodium

Cromolyn sodium is a medication used primarily by patients who have asthma. It is taken by inhalation and works only to *prevent* bronchospasm.

To do so, it must be taken regularly. It should never be used during an asthmatic attack because it actually can make an attack worse.

Expectorants

Expectorants are intended to liquefy secretions and make them easier to cough up. Their value is debated, with no conclusive medical opinion as to whether they work or not. The most widely  used expectorants are potassium iodide (SSKI) and glyceryl guaiacolate (GG). Potassium iodide can cause a rash and swelling of the salivary glands because of allergies to iodide.

Antibiotics

Antibiotic medications are used to fight bacterial infections. Many different types fight different bacteria. Some are given as pills or capsules; others are administered by injection. Penicillin, sulfa drugs, and tetracycline are the generic names 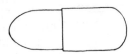 of the most commonly used drugs in this category. You should take these drugs in the exact dose and at the time specified by your doctor, who will tell you what side effects may occur. For example, an upset stomach or bowel problems are rather frequent with certain antibiotics. You must always *finish* the course of antibiotic therapy that your physician prescribes, even though you may feel better after only a few doses.

Diuretics (Water Pills)

Diuretics help rid your body of excess fluid. This fluid, called edema, usually shows up as swollen ankles and legs. There are a number of reasons why edema may develop in patients with lung disease. Diuretics need not be taken if only a little edema occurs in the ankles, but your doctor will make that decision. Overuse of diuretics can make you weak and should be avoided (see the section on potassium supplements).

Digitalis

Digitalis is the generic, overall name for heart pills that strengthen the heart muscle. These drugs make the heart beat slower and with more force. Most patients with lung disease do not have heart problems that require digitalis, but some do. Digitalis drugs must be used carefully. The dose should never be changed without your doctor's order to do so.

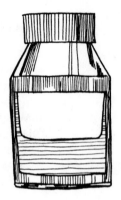

Potassium Supplements

When diuretics are taken regularly, not only fluid but also potassium is lost. This may result in weakness and leg cramps. Potassium supplements are given to counteract these effects. Eating high-potassium foods is sometimes sufficient to replenish lost potassium (see Chapter 12).

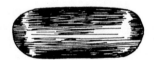

Mood Elevators

Mood elevating drugs are designed to help you feel less depressed.

Tranquilizers and Sedatives

Tranquilizers and sedatives are designed to calm or relax you and to help you sleep. These drugs can dangerously depress your breathing if taken in excess. Therefore the dose should never be increased without consulting your doctor—no matter how nervous or tense you are. Such symptoms (for instance, insomnia or irritability) may mean that your lungs are not working properly and that sedatives and tranquilizers should be decreased, not increased. Your physician knows which medications are best for you.

Flu and Pneumonia Vaccines

Vaccines help you to fight off serious viral (flu) infections and certain other (pneumococcal) infections. A new flu vaccine is prepared each year and usually is available in the fall—before the start of the flu season. The pneumococcal vaccine needs to be given only once.

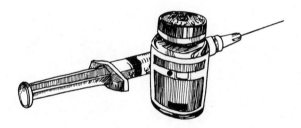

Oxygen

Sometimes patients with lung disease cannot transfer enough oxygen from the alveoli to the blood; therefore the amount of oxygen in the blood falls below normal levels. Such a low blood oxygen level impairs the body's engine (see Chapter 2). People with perfectly normal lungs have the same problem at high altitudes (or when they become astronauts and want to walk around on the moon, where the atmosphere contains no oxygen!). Whatever the reason for the oxygen lack, the treatment is the same: take a drug that overcomes the deficiency. In the case of oxygen deficit that "drug" is oxygen.

Like all drugs, oxygen must be prescribed by your doctor and used with great care. The drugs you take for your respiratory problem are ordered by your doctor in a specific amount, at specific times, to be taken by a specific route. For example, aminophylline (drug), 250 mg. (dose), four times a day (times), by mouth (route). Likewise, oxygen is prescribed by your doctor in the same manner: oxygen (drug), 2 liters/minute (dose), during exercise (times), by nasal cannula (route). Your doctor decides on the appropriate dose based on blood oxygen measurements taken while you rest and exercise. As with other drugs, the dosage of oxygen must not be increased or decreased without the doctor's advice. Turning the liter flow above the prescribed dose may cause serious complications—too much oxygen can injure your lungs and can make your breathing worse. (See Chapter 5 for more information on the use of oxygen.)

•   •   •

Remember that millions of dollars each year are spent on medicines. You can help make the most of your medicine dollar by taking your medications as prescribed by your physician. Each person should receive those medicines that are best for him or her. Those which are good for you may not necessarily be good for your friend or relative!

__ 5

Breathing Paraphernalia

Most people with COPD sooner or later are treated with some type of respiratory therapy equipment or hear about such equipment from others. Often it is first used during a hospitalization and you are not certain why it was used or whether it might be useful at home.

Many ingenious kinds of respiratory therapy equipment have been developed for use by people with COPD. The equipment varies widely in complexity, cost, and usefulness. The device that gave you so much relief in the hospital or in the doctor's office may present many problems for you at home and may not be of value there. Often you can do things yourself that will help your breathing more than any machine! There is no substitute for being informed about your disease.

If you do need equipment at home, the simplest device that will do the job is the best choice. **Remember: The more complex the equipment, the bigger your commitment is for its use, care, and maintenance.** To achieve maximum benefits you should clearly understand the purpose and correct usage of the equipment prescribed for you.

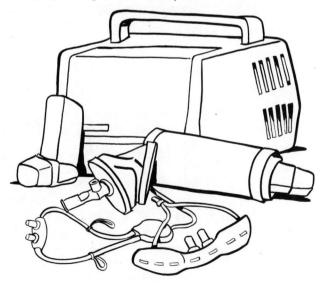

Also, be aware that cost is not a good measure of the value of a device. Inexpensive devices are often as effective as costly ones. Fancy dials and gadgets are no indication that you are getting "the best."

Your doctor should be familiar with these devices and will indicate whether you need them and which best suits your condition.

The devices most frequently used for home care can be conveniently grouped into two categories—oxygen therapy and aerosol therapy. We shall describe the equipment associated with the delivery of oxygen as *oxygen therapy equipment* and the devices that produce visible mist for inhalation as *aerosol therapy equipment*. You may also receive a combination of these treatments.

Oxygen Therapy

What is oxygen? Oxygen is an element, a drug, and a gas. Every cell in the body needs energy to function. Cells get their energy from a combination of the food we eat *plus* oxygen. This energy enables us to use our muscles to breathe, to perform work, and to carry out all bodily functions.

The process by which the body takes in oxygen and eliminates carbon dioxide is called gas exchange (see Chapter 2). If gas exchange does not occur normally, then the oxygen in your blood will be decreased. This is determined by an arterial blood test. If necessary, your doctor will prescribe supplemental oxygen for you (see Chapter 4).

Oxygen makes up 21% of the air around us. This oxygen can be extracted from the air by a very special industrial process that yields 100% oxygen that has been purified and dehumidified. Now the oxygen is ready for packaging and home deliveries.

Today a wide variety of systems are available for home use. Oxygen can be purchased as compressed gas or as a liquid. You can also purchase or

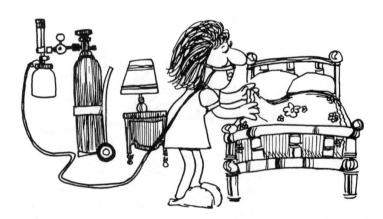

rent electrical devices that generate oxygen from room air. These are called oxygen "concentrators." Some oxygen systems are portable; some are not. The selection of oxygen sources to choose from is broader than ever before and is improving yearly.

Oxygen Equipment

Sources of oxygen

There are three sources of oxygen available for use in the home: compressed gas, liquid oxygen, and oxygen concentrators.

COMPRESSED GAS: TANKS AND CYLINDERS

This is the oldest method for storing oxygen. The oxygen gas is compressed and stored in tanks or cylinders constructed of either steel or aluminum. Aluminum tanks tend to be lighter in weight and more portable. Tanks come in many sizes. Larger stationary ones are often placed in the bedroom; smaller ones are used when exercising or traveling outside the home. For safety reasons, cylinders must be secured upright in a stand or a cart.

LIQUID OXYGEN

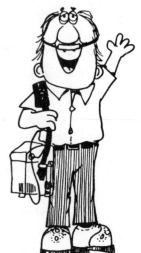

Liquid oxygen is widely used by people who lead active life-styles. It is made through a cooling process that changes the oxygen from a gas to a liquid. The advantage of liquid oxygen is its increased storage capacity. Liquid oxygen can be stored in smaller, more convenient containers than can compressed gas. However, it cannot be stored for long periods of time because it evaporates. Liquid oxygen also requires care in handling.

OXYGEN CONCENTRATOR

An oxygen concentrator is a system for oxygen delivery that is useful for some people. This device is an electrical unit that may resemble a nightstand or end table. It "makes its own oxygen" by "concentrating" the oxygen already present in the air around us. Advantages of this method of oxygen therapy are that it may be less expensive, does not require refilling or replacement of tanks or cylinders, and is easier to manage. However, there are also disadvantages. It is not portable; it may increase your electric bill (even though most gas and electric companies offer a reduced rate for life-supporting equipment, provided you register with them); it may be noisy and give off heat; and back-up cylinders are required in the event of a power failure.

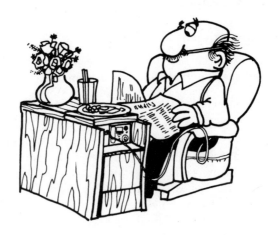

Safety and storage

Oxygen is a relatively safe gas, but because it supports combustion, it must be handled with caution. Oxygen itself does not burn, but it aids in igniting combustible materials. For example, any spark or open flame expands considerably like a "flash fire." Also, oxygen in tanks is under high pressure; therefore, if the top of the tank is knocked loose, the tank can take off like a rocket. Liquid oxygen is very cold, and touching the "steam" that may escape can burn you.

Remember

- The room in which oxygen is stored should be dry, cool, and well ventilated; keep oxygen away from heat, flame, and spark sources.
- Be certain that the oxygen is fastened securely. This will prevent it from being knocked over.
- Avoid inhaling irritating debris that may accumulate at the bottom of cylinders by always changing them when the pressure regulator reads 500 pounds per square inch (psi).
- Never permit grease, oil, or any other potentially combustible substance to come into contact with oxygen-delivery equipment.

- Smoking is not permitted within 10 feet of a source from which oxygen is being administered. Also, there must be at least 10 feet between the oxygen source and any open flame or possible source of electrical sparks.

Oxygen-Delivery Devices

Nasal cannula

Most commonly, a nasal cannula is the appliance used to deliver low concentrations of oxygen for extended periods. The cannula is a light plastic device with two small extensions; one enters each nostril. The cannula is kept in place by an elastic band or lightweight earpiece.

Transtracheal catheter

Transtracheal oxygen is a relatively new method for delivering oxygen in a more efficient and comfortable manner. The catheter is placed directly into the windpipe (trachea) through a small incision in the neck. This is usually done through a minor surgical procedure at an outpatient clinic. Because the oxygen is delivered directly into the lungs, rather than through the nose, the flow rate of oxygen can frequently be reduced; this allows the oxygen source to last for a longer period of time, a distinct advantage for portable systems. In addition, bet-

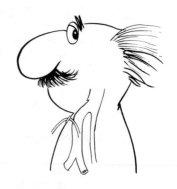

ter oxygenation can be achieved for individuals who require large flow rates. Other possible advantages include more continuous therapy (the catheter stays in place at all times), more comfort and convenience, better cosmetics, and fewer problems related to the nasal cannula on your face. However, use of the transtracheal catheter also requires regular care and cleaning and more problem solving by the patient. Appropriate training in its care needs to be provided.

Oxygen-conserving devices

In addition to transtracheal oxygen therapy, other new devices have been developed to reduce the oxygen-flow requirement and extend the period of time a particular gas source will last. "Reservoir" nasal cannulae provide for storage of oxygen during exhalation in reservoirs located either around the

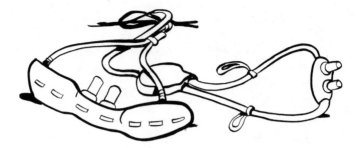

nasal catheter or in a pendant located around the neck. Other devices, called "demand" devices, attach to the oxygen source and turn the flow of oxygen *on* with inspiration (when you "demand" it) and *off* with expiration so that less oxygen is wasted.

Additional Equipment for Oxygen Therapy

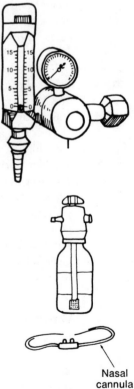

A compressed-gas cylinder has a regulator and flowmeter attached to it. The regulator is a device that reduces the high pressure of the oxygen as it leaves the cylinder. A dial on the regulator also tells you how much oxygen is in the cylinder: a full tank of oxygen usually contains 2200 psi pressure. As you use oxygen, the pressure reading of the cylinder decreases. If you use liquid oxygen, the contents are determined by weighing the container with a scale that comes with that container.

The *flowmeter* is a measuring device or dial; it is part of the oxygen regulator or is attached to your liquid-oxygen container or concentrator. Never use oxygen without a flow control. The flowmeter regulates how much oxygen is delivered to you in liters per minute (see Chapter 4). This is determined and prescribed for you by your doctor.

A *humidifier* is a bottle or jar filled with water and attached to an oxygen flowmeter. The purpose of the humidifier is to replace water vapor that has been removed from oxygen during the process of manufacturing.

Nasal
cannula

Myths and Truths About Oxygen

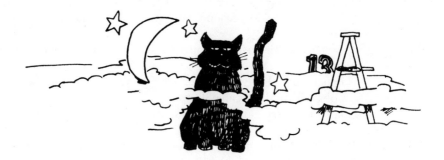

Myth: Oxygen is addicting. Once you start it, you will have to use it forever.

Truth: Oxygen is not addicting. You need use it only when your own lungs cannot supply enough. When you no longer need it, you can stop it.

Myth: If a little oxygen is good, a lot of oxygen is better.

Truth: Oxygen is a drug. Use it only as instructed. Like any drug, too much can be injurious.

Myth: Shortness of breath means lack of oxygen, so if you become short of breath, you should take oxygen.

Truth: Shortness of breath is not always associated with lack of oxygen. If oxygen lack is not the cause, taking oxygen will do no good. Your doctor can do tests to determine whether you need oxygen by taking blood from an artery and measuring the amount of oxygen (arterial blood gas).

Myth: People who need to use oxygen must be confined to their home and can't do anything.

Truth: People who use oxygen can lead a normal life. Several types of portable oxygen systems are available. With good prior planning, you can be active and mobile. Using portable oxygen is not that different from using a hearing aid or glasses—it's just bulkier.

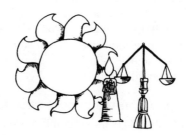

Think Ahead: Questions to Ask
Before You Select a Home Oxygen System

1. Ask your doctor to recommend a practical system for your needs and life-style.
2. Ask your doctor to refer you to a reputable medical equipment supplier.
3. Compare portable systems for cost, weight, size, duration of oxygen supply, and refilling capabilities.
4. Compare oxygen generators for size, noise levels, and monthly electrical cost.
5. Find out whether the system you selected is approved by your medical insurance carrier and whether they will reimburse you for all or part of the cost.
6. Obtain written instructions from your physician or equipment supplier for the correct use of your oxygen system. Make sure you understand these instructions.
7. Learn how to determine the number of hours of oxygen each cylinder will provide. Keep enough on hand. Arrange deliveries on a regular schedule so that you won't run out at night or during a weekend.
8. Ask a family member or friend to assist you in making the equipment selection and in learning about its use and safety.

Aerosol Therapy Devices

The respiratory therapy devices discussed here are those associated with aerosol or "mist" therapy. This treatment modality involves the inhalation of medications and/or water directly into the air passages of the lungs. Inhaling medications is a relatively fast and reliable method for symptom relief. Chest congestion with thick secretions and an ineffective cough can often be relieved with the inhalation of medications and water.

Metered dose inhaler (MDI)

This is a simple, easy-to-handle, and convenient mode for the inhalation of medications. It consists of a small cartridge containing various types of medicine, chiefly bronchodilators or steroids (see Chapter 4), and a mouthpiece for dispensing the drug. The advantage of this type of aerosol therapy is its portability and minimal care, as well as its quick action. Using your MDI requires coordination and timing.

INSTRUCTIONS FOR METERED DOSE INHALER (MDI)

1. Assemble the MDI for use and shake well.
2. Exhale to a comfortable level through pursed lips (see Chapter 6).

3. Place the open end of the mouthpiece slightly in front of your open mouth as shown in the figure at the right.

4. *Do not* close your lips—this allows more air to be inhaled through the mouth to aid in carrying the medication deeper into air passages.

5. As you begin a slow deep breath, press down firmly on the cartridge to release the medication.

6. Hold your breath a few seconds to allow the medication to settle on the surface of your airways. (This will prevent you from exhaling the medication and will aid in obtaining relief.)

7. Exhale slowly and comfortably, using pursed lips.

8. Repeat only as prescribed; rest a few minutes before using again.

9. Keep the MDI clean and free from dirt, lint, and so on by keeping the lid in place.

10. Wash and disinfect the plastic mouthpiece dispenser *regularly* (at least weekly).

11. If you use inhaled steroids, be certain to rinse your mouth after *each use.*

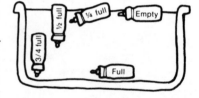

12. Periodically check the amount of medication in your MDI so that you may obtain refills ahead of time. An easy way to estimate how much medication is left inside is to place the cartridge in a container of water and observe its position as it floats.

NOTE: *Do not overuse. Use only as directed by your doctor. Overusing your MDI can result in a rapid, strong heart beat and nervousness.*

Spacers and extenders

Spacers and extenders are chambers placed between you and your metered dose inhaler. They allow the medication to be released first into the chamber and then inhaled 2 to 3 seconds later. The primary advantage is to sim-

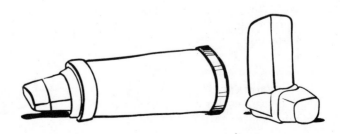

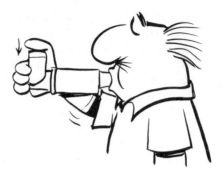

plify the *timing* of medication release, which is so important in using the metered dose inhalers. Spacers and extenders may also help those individuals who experience coughing spasms when using their inhaler. In addition, they help to deliver more of the medication into the lungs and less into the mouth and throat. If your physician prescribes a spacer or extender for you, make sure that you receive instructions for replacement, care, and cleaning of the device.

Nebulizers—the mini-neb and the ultrasonic

A nebulizer is a device that is designed to produce a mist or fog from a liquid; it can be powered either by pressurized air, by oxygen, or by an electrical source.

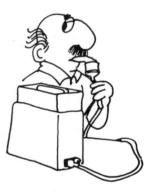

A very popular setup for aerosol therapy at home is the "mini-neb" and air compressor. This system is compact, is simple to operate, and requires little maintenance. It is used primarily to deliver medications or moisture for short periods of time, intermittently throughout the day. The maximum capacity of a small nebulizer is approximately 15 ml (1 tablespoon).

The ultrasonic nebulizer is a very effective nebulizer that operates from an electrical or battery source. Unlike the above-mentioned nebulizers, this unit transforms electrical energy into vibrations, which are then transferred to a liquid. Vibration of the liquid results in a fine, dense, cool mist. This device is more expensive than conventional nebu-

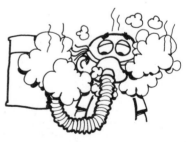

lizers, may require more maintenance, and should be considered for home use only when other aerosol devices do not yield the desired results.

Everything you ever wanted to know about aerosol therapy but were afraid to ask

1. The name of the equipment you are using and its parts
2. How often you should use it (for example, twice a day), and for how long (for example, 20 minutes)
3. What solutions to put in the nebulizer
4. How to prepare, store, and measure the solutions you are using
5. What parts of the nebulizer unit should be removed for cleaning
6. How to clean and disinfect your nebulizer (must be done every 24 hours)
7. How to troubleshoot minor malfunctions
8. **Most important:** the correct breathing pattern to use while taking aerosol therapy; we recommend slow, deep breathing and a slight pause after full inspiration to allow the liquid particles to settle in the lungs

Care and Cleaning of Your Respiratory Equipment

You must take proper care of all equipment that delivers mists or medications into your lungs. If your equipment is contaminated with bacteria, even your own bacteria, you can reinfect yourself and put an extra strain on your lungs and heart. Be sure you clearly understand what equipment parts need to be washed and disinfected. Ask your doctor, therapist, or equipment rental company to recommend an effective technique and disinfecting agent. (We recommend daily cleaning for any mist-producing equipment.)

The following instructions offer a simple approach that is frequently used.

Supplies needed

Liquid detergent (such as Joy)
White vinegar or commercially available disinfectant
Soft brush
Two basins (Do not use sink.)

1. Basin 1 should contain detergent water (discard daily).
2. Basin 2 should hold one part vinegar to one part water (discard every other day; cover between use). If other disinfectants are used, they should be mixed and discarded according to the manufacturer's instruction.

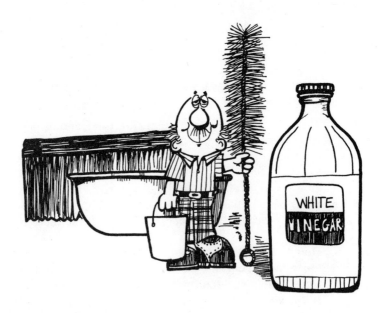

The routine for cleaning

1. Remove all washable parts of equipment and disassemble.
2. Wash in warm water with detergent (basin 1). Scrub all parts gently with brush. Get into all crevices to remove medications, secretions, or any foreign material.
3. Rinse thoroughly under running tap water.
4. Soak equipment in disinfecting solution (basin 2) for a minimum of 30 minutes if using vinegar or according to manufacturer's instructions if using another disinfectant (to kill bacteria). Be sure hollow parts are filled with solution and equipment is completely submerged.
5. Rinse completely under hot tap water; be careful not to touch the sink with your equipment.
6. Air-dry your equipment by:
   a. Shaking or swinging excess water out of tubing and hard-to-dry areas of accessories.
   b. Hanging tubing to allow to drip dry completely
   c. Placing all other pieces of equipment on clean paper towels and covering with paper towels

Remember

1. Discard detergent solution (basin 1) daily.
2. Vinegar solution (basin 2) should be covered and can be kept for 2 days, but no longer. Store in a clean area.

3. Wipe down all surfaces of the machine with a clean damp cloth daily. Then cover and store in a clean area between treatments.
4. Use scrub brush and basins only for equipment cleaning.
5. Store dry tubing and accessories in unused sealed plastic bags.
6. Have two complete sets of washable equipment so you always have a clean, dry set-up available for use the following day.
7. Hair dryers or blowers are not to be used to dry equipment.

All equipment must be washed as stated every 24 hours!

How to prepare sterilized water or normal saline for home use

Here are instructions for making your own solutions for inhalation. Many times it is easier and less expensive for you to prepare them. Remember that bacteria can grow in your solutions unless you are extremely careful! Please follow these instructions exactly as they are written.

1. You need a jar with a lid that fits snugly. A small jam jar or juice bottle will do.
2. Thoroughly wash this jar and its lid in detergent; rinse.
3. Place the jar and its lid in a pan and fill with tap water so that the jar is completely submerged. Place a lid on the pan and gently boil the jar for 15 minutes to sterilize it.
4. After you have boiled the jar, pour the tap water out of the pan. (Use the pan lid to prevent the sterilized jar from falling out.)
5. After the jar and lid have cooled, remove them from the pan. Place them upright on a clean counter. Do not let anything "unsterile" touch the insides of the jar or lid. Do not dry them with a towel or place them upside down to drain.
6. Resterilize the jar and lid at least once each week.
7. Pour distilled water (twice the desired amount) into the clean pan used to boil the jar. If preparing normal saline (salt water), add ¼ teaspoon of salt to every 2 cups of distilled water.
8. Boil gently for 15 minutes. You will have about half the water you started with. Let the water cool and then pour it into the "sterile" jar; cover with lid.

9. Store this in the refrigerator; discard any unused solutions at least once a week.
10. To remove any solution from the jar, pour directly into your nebulizer. Never place an "unsterilized" eyedropper, teaspoon, or other measuring device into the solution in the jar. Do not pour any extra solution back into the jar once it has been removed—discard it.

6

The Art of Better Breathing and Coughing

Breathing Exercises

Pursed lip breathing

The pursed lip breathing technique will aid you in removing trapped air from your lungs and reducing your shortness of breath. In COPD, airways can collapse when you exhale and trap stale air in the air sacs. When this happens, there is not enough room for you to breathe in fresh

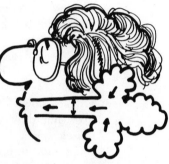

air. Pursed lip breathing provides a resistance to exhaled air at the mouth level and maintains a higher pressure in the airways. This keeps the airways open longer so that more air can get out.
1. Inhale through your nose with your mouth closed.
2. Exhale through your mouth with your lips pursed. (Pursed lips means having your lips in a whistling or kissing position.)
3. Make your exhalation at least twice as long as your inhalation (for example, 2 seconds in, 4 seconds out).

You may want to spend more time breathing out (for example, 2 seconds in, 6 seconds out). Don't force air out to the point of discomfort.

Pursed lip breathing is a basic technique used with all other breathing exercises and physical activities. When you become short of breath, it should be practiced along with diaphragmatic breathing. Learn it first and learn it well.

Diaphragmatic breathing

Normal movement of the diaphragm

The diaphragmatic breathing exercise will reactivate and strengthen the diaphragm. Normally the diaphragm does about 80% of the work of breathing. In COPD the diaphragm flattens and the upper chest mus-

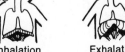

Inhalation   Exhalation

cles try to take over. These muscles require more energy and oxygen to do the diaphragm's job. To locate your diaphragm, place your flat hand on the center of your stomach at the base of the breastbone—then sniff. You will feel your diaphragm move.

EXERCISE 1—FRONT EXPANSION

Assume a comfortable position as indicated in the picture.

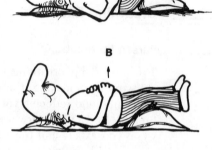

1. Place one hand in the center of your stomach at the base of your breastbone—this hand will detect the movement of your diaphragm.
2. Place your other hand on your upper chest—this hand will detect the movement of the upper chest and accessory muscles (which you want to deemphasize).
3. Exhale slowly through pursed lips while drawing your stomach muscles inward (Figure A).
4. Inhale slowly through your nose—your stomach should expand outward (Figure B). The hand over the diaphragm should feel the most movement.
5. Rest.

Exercise 2—lower side rib breathing

Assume a comfortable sitting or standing position and good posture.

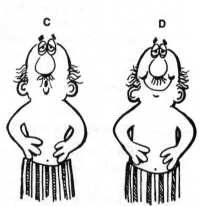

1. Place your hands on your sides at the base of your ribs.
2. Breathe out slowly through pursed lips. Your ribs should move inward (Figure C).
3. Breathe in slowly through the nose and allow ribs to expand outward against your hands (Figure D).
4. Rest.

After you have mastered each of these exercises, practice combining them.

It is necessary to practice often to

strengthen and coordinate your muscles. Set aside certain times (two or three) throughout the day to practice. Be sure to rest after three or four deep breaths to avoid becoming lightheaded. Concentrate on making each breath slow and deep. Pursed lip breathing should always be used when practicing diaphragmatic breathing.

Diaphragmatic breathing can become your normal breathing pattern if practiced faithfully and will result in less shortness of breath. Whenever you become short of breath, diaphragmatic and pursed lip breathing should be used. They should also be used during exercise and during strenuous activities. You must master these techniques before going on to other exercises.

Controlled Coughing Technique

Coughing is the natural way of removing foreign substances from the lungs. In COPD there is often an excess production of mucus, which must be removed to maintain open airways and allow you to move air in and out of your lungs effectively. If the excess mucus is not removed, shortness of breath can worsen. Retained mucus can also contribute to the risk of infection. In addition, the mucus irritates nerve endings in the tracheobronchial tree and can cause frequent, involuntary coughing, resulting in fatigue. To conserve energy and oxygen, you must practice and master the method of controlled coughing.

STEP 1. Take a slow deep breath, using diaphragmatic breathing. Building up a volume of air behind the mucus helps to propel it toward the mouth.

STEP 2. Hold the deep breath for 2 seconds.

STEP 3. Cough twice with your mouth slightly open. The first cough loosens and the second cough moves the mucus.

STEP 4. Pause.

STEP 5. Inhale by sniffing gently. Taking in a big breath after coughing only causes you to cough again and may drive the mucus back into the lungs.

STEP 6. Rest.

A drink of water taken before coughing can be helpful. Coughing is easier when you are in a sitting position with your head slightly forward and your feet supported. Controlled, effective coughing should make a hollow sound.

Coughing Steps in Brief

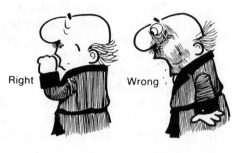

Right   Wrong

1. Deep breath.
2. Hold your breath.
3. Cough twice.
4. Pause.
5. Inhale by sniffing gently.
6. Rest.

If you need to cough again, repeat the procedure step by step.

Control your cough—don't let it control you!

7

Day In, Day Out: Your Daily Activities

The use of proper breathing techniques while going about your daily routine will enable you to do *more* with *less* shortness of breath. You must pace your work to your capacity and always maintain a controlled breathing pattern. If you feel like taking a couple of breaths between the work, do so— then continue as described. It is not necessary to work on every exhalation.

Rules

1. Take a deep breath by using your diaphragm before doing any work (especially something strenuous).
2. While you are exhaling (which is the most passive part of breathing), the work itself should be performed.
3. Remember to breathe out at least twice as long as you breathe in (for example, inhale 2 seconds, exhale 4 seconds).

Standing up from a chair

Take a deep breath by using your diaphragm.
While breathing out through pursed lips, rise to your feet.

Going up a flight of stairs or walking up a hill

Take a deep breath by using your diaphragm before you start to climb.
   While breathing out through pursed lips, climb two or three stairs or take two or three steps.
Stop and rest while breathing in with your diaphragm again.
If you should feel short of breath at this point, rest for a while, taking as many breaths as you need to feel comfortable again. Then continue climbing in the same manner as just described.

Lifting loads

Take a deep breath by using your diaphragm.

Bend at the hips and knees and not at the waist. Hold the load close to your body.

While breathing out with pursed lips, lift and place load where intended. Keep your back rounded as you return to standing.

Many people with COPD regard all arm movements, especially about the shoulders, as difficult and tiresome. The following examples show you how to coordinate proper breathing with these movements.

Pushing a broom, vacuum cleaner, or lawn mower

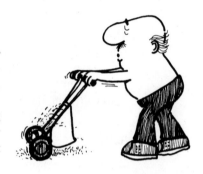

Take a deep breath by using your diaphragm before you start to push.

Push objects while breathing out with pursed lips.

Stop and rest while breathing in, using your diaphragm again. Continue your pushing in the same manner as just described.

Shaving, combing hair

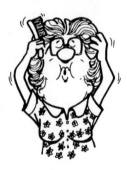

Take a deep breath by using your diaphragm.

While breathing out with pursed lips, lift your arms and shave or comb two or three strokes.

Lower your arms and rest while breathing in, using your diaphragm again.

Continue your shaving or combing in the same manner as just described.

Reaching

Take a deep breath by using your diaphragm.

While breathing out with pursed lips, lift your arms to shoulder level or above, reaching for the intended goal.

Some additional examples of when you might use this breathing technique

Household Tasks
Bedmaking
Window washing
Mopping
Moving furniture
Putting away dishes

Garden Work
Digging
Raking leaves
Weeding

Exercises	Hobbies
Walking	Golfing
Arm exercises	Bowling
Breathing exercises	
Body improvement exercises	**Personal Hygiene**
Bronchial drainage	Dressing
Relaxation exercises	Brushing Teeth
	Showering

Some Examples of Energy-Saving Techniques

Economizing your energy can be important to complete your necessary daily chores. Often this can be accomplished by slight changes in the way you perform these tasks.

1. Plan your daily chores in advance so you won't feel rushed or have to push beyond your limitations.
2. Decide which jobs are absolutely necessary to make your home comfortable and attractive.
3. Adopt a cooperative work-sharing attitude within your family. Assign tasks and responsibilities.
4. Pace all work to your own speed.
5. Distribute tedious tasks throughout the week.
6. Do the tasks requiring the most exertion when you have the most energy. For example, if mornings are difficult, take your shower and set the breakfast table the evening before.
7. Interchange the easy activities with the difficult ones, and take rest periods in between to prevent overfatigue.
8. When possible, sit down to work. For example, make use of a kitchen stool and a shower stool.
9. Drain dishes dry instead of towel drying.

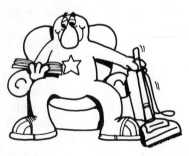

10. Prepare food for two or more meals at one cooking session. Refrigerate or freeze the additional meals for another time.
11. Unclutter your storage areas (such as cupboards, wardrobes, and tool sheds) so that you can easily find and reach what you need.
12. Avoid ironing clothes as much as possible by using drip-dry or permanent-press fabrics.
13. Straighten up rooms as you go along. A good rule is "never leave a room empty handed."
14. Vacuuming may leave fine dust in the air. To prevent breathing it, tie a moist handkerchief in front of your mouth and nose while vac-

uuming; open windows and let the room air out for at least an hour. Use only disposable vacuum bags.

15. When making your bed, start at the head and progress down the bed toward and across the foot, tucking in and smoothing as you go. Then proceed up the second side. A bed on casters makes moving it easier; however, it is more convenient if only the head of the bed is against the wall. Because an electric blanket is light weight, it is easier to lift and weighs less heavily on your body at night.

Some Tips for Daily Self-Care

Your hygiene and grooming can be some of the more exerting activities you have to perform in a day.

1. Caring for the hair is less work if you have a short, easy-to-maintain haircut.

2. If brushing teeth is a chore, use an electric toothbrush.

3. If you feel smothered under an overhead shower or when splashing water on your face, use a washcloth and install a hand shower to control the direction and force of flow.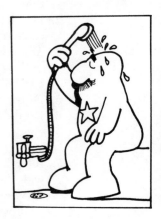

4. If steam in the shower bothers you, try turning on the cold water first, then slowly add the hot. (Don't forget to use a stool to sit on while in the shower!)

5. Putting grab bars and no-slip strips in the tub or shower will help you keep your balance.

6. Avoid all scented soaps, colognes, and other grooming products if you find they bother your breathing.

7. To scrub your back, use a folded towel with handles at each end and with a brush or loofah sponge attached in the middle; this is easy to pull diagonally back and forth across your back. These are available in most bath shops.

8. Rubbing yourself dry after a bath can be very tiring. Try wrapping yourself in a terry cloth robe. Its absorbent qualities will dry you "automatically."

9. Be sure to use your oxygen in the shower or bath if you have been prescribed oxygen with activity. The portable tank can be set just outside the shower or tub and extra-long tubing used.

10. Do not "lock yourself up" in the bathroom. Keep windows and doors open as much as possible. Otherwise, use a fan. The air does

not necessarily have to be fresh for you to breathe better, as long as it circulates.

• • •

Remember, coordinate your breathing techniques with all of these activities:

1. Use the diaphragm and relax the accessory muscles when you breathe in.
2. Purse your lips while you breathe out; breathe out at least twice as long as you breathe in.
3. Do strenuous work—especially work involving climbing, holding the arms up, and compressing the trunk—on exhalation only.

__8

Cleaning Out Your Tubes: Bronchial Drainage

Many persons with chronic lung disease have secretions in their bronchial tubes that not only make it more difficult to breathe but also may interfere with oxygen getting into the blood. These secretions are also a perfect place for bacteria to grow, multiply, and cause a major lung infection. By draining these secretions, you will be able to breathe more easily, prevent infections, and generally feel better.

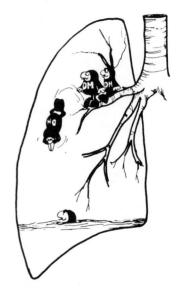

Secretions tend to pool in the bottom of your lungs because humans spend most of their time in the upright position. To get secretions to a point where you can cough them up more easily, you must tilt your chest so that, with the assistance of gravity, the bronchial tubes of the lower lung area can drain; this is bronchial drainage.

You should learn techniques of bronchial drainage from a therapist or nurse only when ordered by your doctor. Some basic points, the steps to follow, and pictures of bronchial drainage positions will help you to remember what you have learned.

BASIC POINTS

- Bronchial drainage is best done first thing in the morning (1 hour before breakfast) and in the evening (at least 1 hour before bedtime).
- Bronchial drainage should be done at least once or twice daily. Increase the number of treatments to three or four when your secretions change color or increase in amount or when you have a cold.

- When you feel like doing your bronchial drainage the least, you probably need it the most.
- It is most important to tilt the chest area 10 to 20 degrees below the horizontal level. This can be accomplished by using one of the following suggested methods:

> A slant board
> Couch pillows placed on the floor
> Firm pillows propped under your hips in bed

There is no excuse for skipping your bronchial drainage!

Steps to Follow for Effective Bronchial Drainage

STEP 1. *Conditioning of airways and secretions*

Take prescribed medications to dilate your airways before you begin bronchial drainage. Oral bronchodilator medicine should ideally be taken at least 30 minutes beforehand. Inhaled bronchodilator medicine should be taken at least 10 minutes before doing bronchial drainage.

Drink at least 1½ quarts of liquid daily. Adequate fluid intake is mandatory to keep mucus thin. Breathe in moist air (from nebulizers, vaporizers, a warm shower, or boiling water placed in a bowl). These techniques also help to make mucus thin.

STEP 2. *Good inflation of the lungs*

Breathing exercises are extremely important. Diaphragmatic and pursed lip breathing should be done throughout the bronchial drainage period. They help widen your airways so secretions can be drained.

STEP 3. *Use of gravity, percussion, and vibration*

The use of gravity is the most important aspect of draining secretions. The positions on the next page show gravity drainage positions. Stay in each of the positions (1 through 4) for 5 to 15 minutes.

Percussion and vibration are additional methods of loosening secretions. Percussion may be prescribed for at least 1 minute in each position. Percussion, or clapping with a cupped hand on the chest wall, helps to move secretions into larger airways. Percussion should be done only on the rib cage and not over the spinal column, breastbone, or soft tissues.

Vibration is the other means of moving secretions. Your rib cage may be vibrated by another person or a mechanical device. Vibration should follow percussion and is done for an additional minute only when you are exhaling.

Your skin should be covered with clothing or a towel during per-

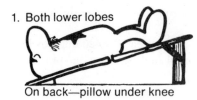

1. Both lower lobes

On back—pillow under knee

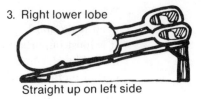

3. Right lower lobe

Straight up on left side

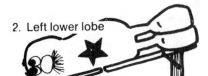

2. Left lower lobe

Straight up on right side

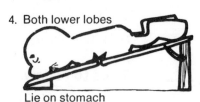

4. Both lower lobes

Lie on stomach

cussion and vibration. Your doctor or therapist should instruct you in these procedures.

If additional positions are needed, your doctor, therapist, or nurse will prescribe them.

STEP 4. *Controlled coughing*

Remember to cough after each position. Use the controlled coughing technique. Rest after coughing.

Precautions

If you have high blood pressure or a heart problem, be sure to check with your doctor before doing bronchial drainage. If you are on steroids or have osteoporosis (weak bones), check with your doctor before doing percussion or vibration on your chest.

Remember these four key steps:
1. Condition airways and secretions.
2. Inflate lungs.
3. Use gravity drainage.
4. Cough after each position.

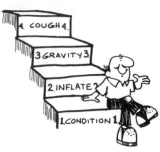

9

The Joy of Exercise

First Things First

Good physical condition is an objective that everyone should seek; the person with COPD is no exception. Individuals with COPD frequently avoid physical activity because of the limitations imposed by shortness of breath. In addition, friends, family, or physicians may have encouraged them not to exert themselves, assuming that to do so might cause "harmful effects." After years of study we now know this isn't true. *Inactivity is an enemy working against you!* Sitting or lying around deconditions the body and makes all of your muscles less strong and less efficient. This in turn makes performing even the simplest daily activities more difficult, energy-wise and breathing-wise. This deconditioning effect can be reversed by a regular exercise program. The three major systems involved in exercise are the skeletal muscles, specialized heart muscles, and respiratory muscles. With progressive exercise of any kind, the fibers of the muscles involved become more efficient; that is, they need less and less oxygen for the same amount of work. Thus you may have more "energy" to accomplish the tasks you perform each day, and you may do these tasks with less shortness of breath.

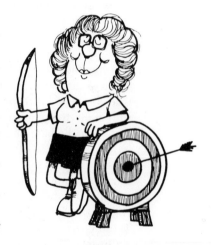

The reconditioning of muscles should be undertaken with great care because suddenly starting to exercise may be useless at best and hazardous at worst. The proper way to approach improving your physical condition depends on two fundamentals:

1. Choosing appropriate goals
2. Your overall health at the time you start a physical conditioning program

Someone whose goal is to win the Olympic mile run and who is 18 years old with no health limitations can follow a program that consists of running more and more miles each week at a faster and faster pace. This program, like all conditioning programs, will be progressive; that is, it will increase in distance and speed until the maximum tolerable level is reached.

Weight lifters, on the other hand, would start a progressive program of muscle building that involves techniques quite unlike those used by a runner. Gymnasts and ballet dancers would also follow different routines. They too need conditioning. But for their goals, different muscles are involved, and they seek body flexibility, as well as endurance and strength. A physical conditioning program designed for a weight lifter might ruin the career of a gymnast or ballet dancer.

Furthermore, a program developed for a young athlete can be hazardous for an individual who has a known (or unknown) health problem. A 50-year-old man who has decided to enter the "Senior Olympics" should devise his physical conditioning program with great caution and under close medical guidance. Otherwise, a heart attack (rather than a new world record) can be his reward. Similar cautions apply to the Sunday tennis player who in 90° temperatures is carried away by the contest, failing to recognize that he or she has not exercised regularly during prior weeks (or months).

So, regardless of the individual involved, the goals of the program and consideration of overall health status should precede the starting of a physical conditioning program.

Like the different types of athletes, people with COPD should set specific goals involving the physical activities that they would like to achieve. These goals should be realistic and, preferably, written down.

In goal setting, the athlete is limited by his natural abilities, body build, and motivation. A 4-foot 10-inch athlete should not aim at being a star professional basketball center. The patient with COPD is also subject to these limitations in goal setting, plus an additional one: the status of his or her lung function. Careful evaluation of the type and extent of lung function abnormalities present is es-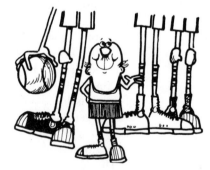sential before establishing a physical conditioning program. Such evaluation is required for the following two reasons:

1. Certain specific physical conditioning techniques can be undertaken in the COPD patient to improve lung function itself.
2. The status of lung function must be known to establish safe limits of exercise.

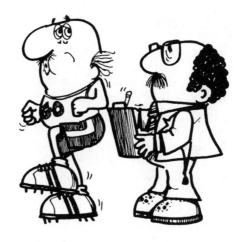

Play It Safe

You should consult your physician before beginning an exercise program. You can then work together in choosing the type of exercise that is most useful and best fits in with your life-style.

Each part of your physical conditioning program should be checked for safety before you attempt it. This is not a responsibility you should assume. For example, walking too far too quickly may put excessive strain on your lungs or heart. Or certain physical activities may cause your blood oxygen level to fall to undesirable levels. Therefore do not attempt to construct your own program. Your doctor will do that with you. Your doctor wants you to be in optimal condition—but within the limits he knows are safe. These limits can be established only by testing, then by tailoring your program to your specific lung, heart, and other limitations. There are no simple guidelines that you yourself can establish. For instance, becoming short of breath during a given exercise does not mean that you are overdoing it and have to stop. If it did, most athletes would stop in the middle of a race, a tennis match, or a football game. Even fatigue or aching muscles do not necessarily mean you are overdoing it. It may be necessary to experience such discomforts to improve your condition. So let your physician set the limits, based on his detailed knowledge of your condition.

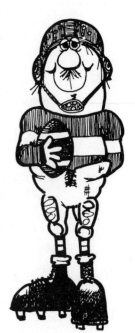

Types of Exercise

The kind of exercise that will benefit you most depends on what you want to do. What does that mean? It means that exercise training is rather specific: weight lifting, swimming, bicycling, running, dancing, jumping, calisthenics, and so on, all "train" different muscles. Most people with COPD want to increase their ability to walk in terms of both speed and distance. In fact, walking is one of the best forms of exercise because: (1) it uses many body muscles, including the heart and diaphragm; (2) it requires no special equipment or skill; and (3) it can be measured easily (for instance, by speed or distance). Therefore, walking is the usual starting point for most people with COPD. From this starting point you may want to branch out to other types of exercise.

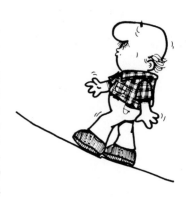

Your Job

Whatever exercise program is designed for you, you will be responsible for mastering it. You will find that you may have to push yourself some to establish a regular routine. Being short of breath creates a big temptation to remain inactive, especially on the days when the shortness of breath may seem worse. When planning a safe exercise schedule remember to start slowly. Plan a progressive walking program beginning with short distances and a slow pace. You may gradually increase the duration of your walks as your strength and endurance increase. Keep a careful record of your exercise sessions—for example, how long you walked, how fast you walked, your pulse rate before and after exercise, and how you tolerated the exercise. Then, you and your doctor can monitor your progress and adjust your exercise routine as necessary.

Your doctor and other health professionals will guide you. But it is your job to pick up the ball and carry through by following the program *regularly*.

10

Letting Go: Relaxation Techniques

Why Talk About Relaxation?

When you are physically and emotionally relaxed, you avoid excessive oxygen consumption caused by tension from overworked muscles. Relaxation also decreases other undesirable manifestations of stress such as mental irritability and anxiety that might induce bronchospasm, increased shortness of breath, and fatigue. By using some of the suggested relaxation methods outlined below, you can relieve the tension that increases your respiratory difficulties. Complete muscular relaxation is also important to gain maximum benefits from all other exercises.

The key to relaxation is, above all, breathing control. When you can master diaphragmatic breathing, relaxation of the accessory muscles, and prolonged exhalation with pursed lips at times of stress, you have achieved a major victory in the battle against panic. At such times also remember positioning, which can be either standing or sitting, but always leaning forward with your arms supported.

To practice this first progressive relaxation technique, lie down on a comfortable surface and place a pillow under your head and knees. Quiet, peaceful surroundings are helpful. The principle that applies here is that maximum relaxation follows maximum contraction. Always tighten and relax the muscles gradually.

HEAD AND NECK

Pull chin down toward chest as tightly as possible and push back of head into pillow, then let go.

Turn head from side to side in a relaxed manner. Let it stop when it comes to a comfortable position.

SHOULDERS

Shrug shoulders and tighten the shoulder muscles as much as possible, then release.

ARMS

Do one hand and one arm at a time.

Bend elbow and make a fist out of your hand. Tighten as much as possible, then let go.

Straighten arm and fingers. Tighten as much as possible, then release.

LEGS

Do one leg at a time.

Straighten leg and point toe; tighten as much as possible, then let go. Pull toes toward your nose, and push heel and back of leg into bed. Tighten as much as possible, then release.

BACK

Arch your back up in the same slow, easy way a cat does. Do not lift your hips while arching. Tighten as much as possible, then let go.

FACE

Tighten (scrinch) all of your face muscles. Hold, then release.

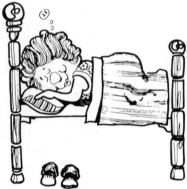

EYES

Try to focus your eyes on something. Watch it and slowly let your eyelids grow heavy. Open your eyes and let them close gradually until they feel comfortable while closed.

Sweet dreams!

Other Relaxation Techniques

Another way to control your tension is to create in your mind a mental picture of something that gives you a good and comfortable feeling. This may be a scene, real or imagined: a landscape with rolling hills; green grass and trees with their leaves gently moving in the wind; the beach; a poolside; or your mother's kitchen. Try to make your mental picture detailed. Each time you find yourself physically in a difficult situation that you cannot immediately leave (for example, a crowded elevator), use the visual image you have created as a mental escape. This will help keep your anxiety and shortness of breath under control until you can physically remove yourself from that situation.

"Mind-over-matter" relaxation techniques are another way to help increase your mind's awareness and control over your body. There are many

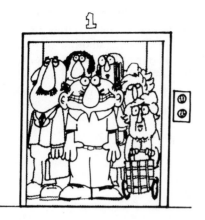 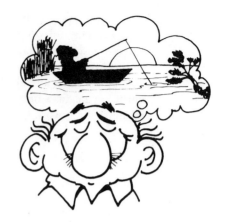

different ways to do this type of "self-hypnosis." You can simply concentrate on a certain part of your body; for instance, concentrate on your right hand and envision that it is becoming very limp, soft, heavy, or light. Any of these sensations will induce relaxation. Sometimes during a stressful or anxiety-provoking event, blood will rush to the center of the body, leaving the limbs cool and moist. Thinking of your hands and feet as "getting warm" is very effective because relaxation occurs when the temperature increases. Try it first with one hand and, when you have succeeded in warming it, proceed up the arm, then to the shoulder, then to the other hand, and so on until you have finally "told" your whole body to relax and it has obeyed you.

Another useful relaxation technique is one most frequently used in different types of meditation. Concentrate on one word and repeat it over and over to yourself (such as the word "free"). Repeat the word each time you breathe out. Do not let yourself be distracted by intruding thoughts; ignore them and return to repeating your word. Don't be concerned about how deep a relaxation level you are reaching. When trying these different modes of relaxation exercises, become passive and allow relaxation to come about at its own pace.

Sleep eradicates the effects of daily fatigue. Many people with COPD, however, have trouble sleeping, sometimes because of their medications. In addition, the events of modern life frequently overload human faculties, causing exhaustion that may not be corrected by sleep. Meditation is thought to produce an extraordinarily deep rest and a stress release much more complete than sleep. It is particularly suited for gradual removal of long-accumulated stress. This may be one relaxation method you might want to investigate further. Meditation can be used in conjunction with the progressive relaxation technique first mentioned. You start by relaxing your muscles, then you meditate.

Other modes of relaxation include learning to give yourself a massage or having your spouse give you one, especially on the neck and shoulder muscles. The vibrator you use for bronchial drainage can be very useful for this purpose also (see Chapter 8). Biofeedback is another way to learn to relax and to explore your own ability to control tension and shortness of breath. You might have already found your own way to relax—for instance, soft music, yoga, or a bubble bath. There are many simple techniques worth trying. If they work for you, use them!

11

Making Your Body Work Better

Body-Improvement Exercises

The techniques described here will not help the lungs themselves but will improve your entire physical condition. These body-improvement exercises will increase the efficiency of your muscles so that they require less fuel (oxygen) during exertion.

Before starting on these exercises, you want to be sure that your lungs are as "clean" as possible. So, if you have excess mucus, you should clear your lungs of mucus by the techniques already described before beginning these exercises. If you are tense, total body–relaxation techniques should be followed before exercise. And if pursed lip breathing or diaphragmatic breathing has been prescribed for you, you should use these methods during exercise.

In other words, you should have "all systems go" before "blasting off" into body-improvement exercises. This is like the athlete who warms up before his event. Once you are warmed up, you can get started!

Each exercise may be performed daily two to ten times after first checking with your physician or therapist regarding your specific physical limitations (see Chapter 9). Start the exercise program by performing only a couple of repetitions of each exercise. Increase the repetitions gradually.

Warm-up exercises to relax shoulder and neck muscles

The shoulder and neck muscles are considered accessory respiratory muscles and are not normally involved in the work of quiet breathing. Some individuals with COPD tend to breathe shallowly, using upper chest muscles because of decreased mobility of the rib cage and flattening of the diaphragm. To breathe properly, you must relax your shoulder and neck muscles. The following exercises can be performed anytime during the day when you feel tense in the shoulder and neck area. They should also be done between the other exercises in your body-improvement program.

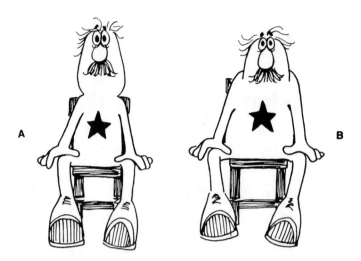

SHOULDER SHRUGGING

1. Stand or sit with feet slightly apart and arms relaxed (Figure A).
2. Shrug shoulders and tighten the muscles as much as possible (Figure B).
3. Relax and rest.
4. Repeat up to ten times.

ELBOW CIRCLING

1. Sit or stand with hands on shoulders.
2. Circle the elbows forward, up, back, and downward. Do two to ten circles.
3. Relax muscles.

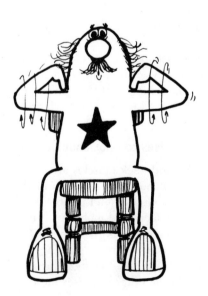

HEAD CIRCLING

1. Roll head slowly from side to side in a forward semicircle.
2. Repeat a couple of times.
3. *Do not* arch your neck by rolling your head back.

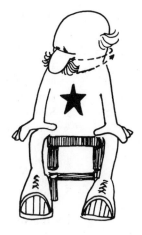

CIRCLING OF SHOULDERS WITH HANGING ARMS

1. Sit or stand with arms relaxed.
2. Circle right shoulder up and back (Figure A).
3. Repeat up to ten times.
4. Repeat on left side.
5. Finally circle both shoulders together (Figure B).
6. Repeat up to ten times.
7. Repeat the exercise in the opposite direction.

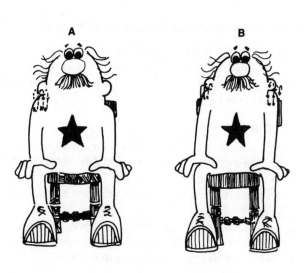

OVER-THE-HEAD SHOULDER STRETCH

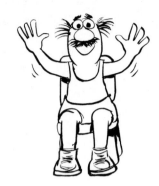

1. Sit and press lower back firmly against back of chair.
2. Pretend you hold a stick. Keep both arms outstretched and 3 feet apart. Do not lock elbows.
3. Slowly raise your extended arms above your head to the place where the top of your shoulders feels tight.
4. Hold the position at the tightest place for 5 to 10 seconds.
5. Return to starting position and relax.

UNDERNEATH SHOULDER STRETCH

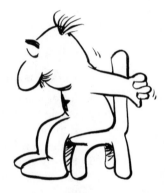

1. Sit and bend your head and chest forward slightly.
2. Reach your arms behind your back, clasp your hands together and lift slowly.
3. Hold the position at the place where the muscles feel the tightest for 5 to 10 seconds.
4. Return to starting position and relax.

   Comments: Do the last two stretching exercises once each. Try to gradually increase the holding time of the stretched position up to the point where you feel a release of the tightness in the muscles.

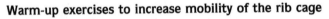

Warm-up exercises to increase mobility of the rib cage

Some individuals with COPD develop stiff rib cages, especially the lower ribs. If this is a problem, the following group of exercises will help to increase the mobility of the rib cage. This enables the lower lung areas to expand more fully.

FORWARD BENDING

1. Sit in a straight-backed chair, feet flat on the floor and slightly apart, shoulders relaxed, arms comfortable at the sides (Figure A).
2. While exhaling, drop your head to your chest and slowly roll your body forward, toward your knees (Figure B). Do *not* jackknife at the waist (Figure C).
3. Return to the upright position slowly by pushing first the lower, then the middle, then the upper back against the chair.
4. Relax, inhale, then repeat up to ten times.

A   B   C

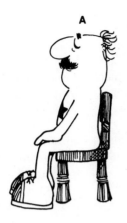
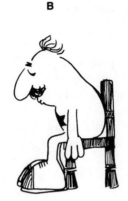
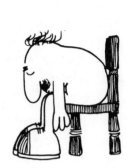

SIDE BENDING

1. Sit up straight with feet apart. Place left hand on lower left rib cage and place right hand on top of left hand.
2. While exhaling slowly, bend head and shoulders to the left while pressing hands against left side (Figure A).
3. Then, while inhaling and in a continuous motion, bend the head and shoulders slightly to the right while expanding the left lower ribs as much as possible (Figure B).
4. Return to starting position and rest.
5. Repeat on the other side.
6. Repeat up to ten times on both sides.

A   B

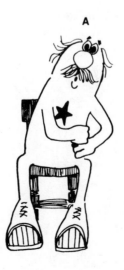
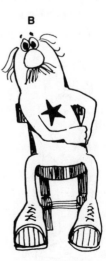

Exercises to improve arm performance

Because arm movement can be very strenuous for individuals with COPD, it is important to maintain muscle strength and endurance with simple arm exercises. Work both arms simultaneously, maintaining the muscle tension as you do each exercise. Do not suddenly relax or drop your arms. Do all arm movements on exhalation only. Try to complete each set on consecutive exhalations.

Initially perform one set of six repetitions of each arm exercise. Rest one minute between each set. As your strength and endurance improve, proceed to two sets of each exercise, using the same weight. Finally, proceed to three sets. Complete the various sets of each exercise consecutively. When you can comfortably do three sets of six lifts of all the arm exercises, you may increase your weights by ½ to 1 pound.

After a weight increase, begin with one set of six lifts of each exercise, gradually progressing to three sets of six lifts of each exercise. Perform your weight-lifting exercise every other day. Do not use weights heavier than four pounds for men and three pounds for women.

During the chair arm exercises, sit with your hip and knee joints at 90-degree angles with feet flat on the floor. Press your lower back firmly against the back of the chair during arm activity. Do not allow an increase in the curvature of your lower back. Lift your arms initially only as far as you can without arching your back. Do not lock your elbows during weight lifting. If pain or other unusual symptoms arise during arm exercise, *stop* the painful motion and *do not repeat it*. Coordinate your breathing with motion. Do not run out of breath before a motion is completed.

DIAGONAL ARM RAISES

1. Sit in a straight-backed chair with your feet slightly apart and your arms crossed in your lap (Figure A).
2. While exhaling, lift your arms upward out in a straight diagonal (Figure B).

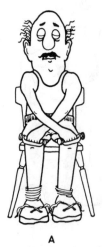   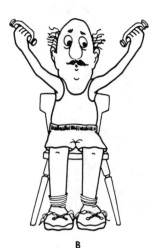   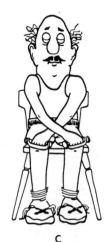

A   B   C

3. On the same exhalation, reverse the motion and return to starting position (Figure C).
4. Repeat six times, then rest.

SIDEWARD ARM RAISES

1. Sit in a straight-backed chair with your feet slightly apart and your arms down at your sides (Figure A).
2. While exhaling, lift arms out and up until they are vertical above the head (Figure B and C).
3. On the same exhalation, reverse motion and return to starting position. (Figure D).
4. Repeat six times, then rest.

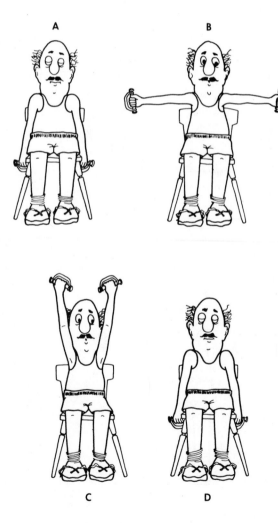

A

B

C

D

SIDE-FORWARD ARM RAISES

1. Sit in a straight-backed chair with your feet slightly apart and your arms down at your sides (Figure A).
2. While exhaling, lift arms out and up to a horizontal position, then forward until hands meet in front of your body (Figures B and C).
3. On the same exhalation, reverse the motion and return to starting position (Figures D and E).
4. Repeat six times, then rest.

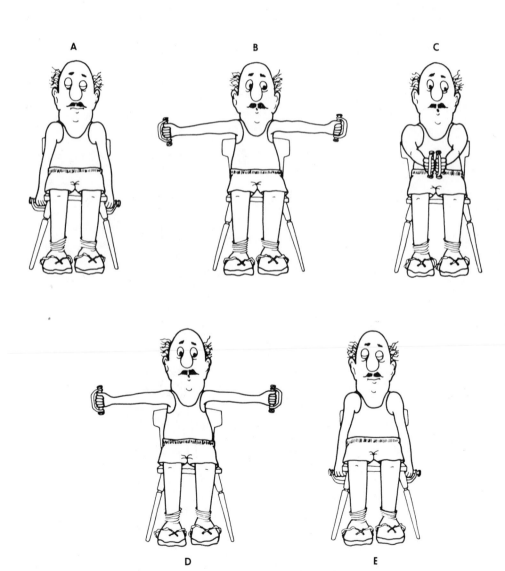

A

B

C

D

E

STRAIGHT ARM RAISES BACKWARD AND FORWARD

1. Lie on your back with knees bent, feet flat on the floor, arms at your sides, and weights in hands (Figure A).
2. Keep the small of your back pressed against the floor.
3. While exhaling, lift straight arms up and back as far as you can without feeling movement in your back (Figures B and C).
4. On the same exhalation, reverse the movement by bringing your straight arms forward and down again by your sides (Figures D and E).
5. Repeat six times, then rest.

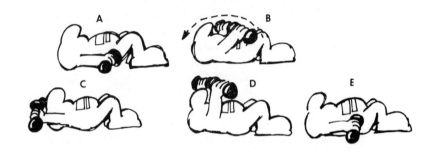

ELBOW BENDS WITH ARMS UP

1. Assume the same starting position as in previous exercise.
2. While exhaling, bend your elbows (Figure A).
3. Keep the small of your back pressed against the floor.
4. On the same exhalation, straighten arms up in the air and return to bent elbows (Figures B and C).
5. Repeat six times, then rest.

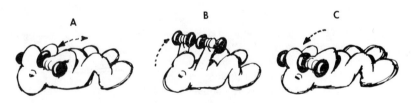

STRAIGHT ARM RAISES INWARD AND OUTWARD

1. Lie with your arms at a 90-degree angle from your body (straight out from your sides).
2. Keep the small of your back pressed against the floor.
3. While exhaling, lift both arms straight up so your hands meet above your face (Figures A and B).
4. Return to the original position on the same exhalation.
5. Repeat six times, then rest.

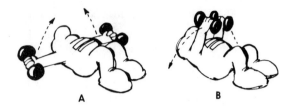

A   B

Exercises to strengthen abdominal muscles

Some people with COPD must work to get air out, as well as in. Strong abdominal muscles can help push air out by compressing the rib cage and pulling the lower ribs downward. Through active exercise, the abdominal muscles can regain their elasticity and their capacity to relax. This aids diaphragmatic breathing, effective coughing, and muscular back support. These exercises must be done smoothly and slowly. You must contract your stomach muscles and press the small of your back against the floor while performing head, shoulder, and leg raises.

CONTRACTION OF ABDOMINAL MUSCLES WITH PELVIC TILT

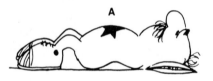

1. Lie on your back with your knees bent and feet flat on the floor. Place a pillow under your head (basic starting position, Figure A).
2. While exhaling, contract the abdominal muscles and roll your hips under so that your back is flat against the floor (Figure B).
3. Relax your muscles and rest.
4. Repeat up to ten times.

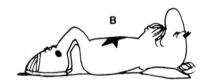

NOTE: *If you are unable to contract your abdominal muscles as described, start your exercise program with any of the following exercises until you gain awareness of the state of your abdominal muscles and how to use them.*

HEAD AND SHOULDER RAISING

1. Assume the basic starting position and cross your arms in front of your chest.
2. With your chin tucked in and while exhaling, raise your head and shoulders.
3. Return to starting position while still exhaling and then rest.
4. Repeat once.

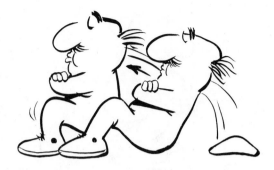

KNEE BENDING

1. Assume the basic starting position shown in Figure A.
2. While exhaling, bring the left knee toward your left shoulder and press the small of your back against the floor (Figure B).
3. Return to starting position and relax.
4. Repeat on right side.
5. Repeat up to ten times on each side.

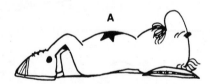
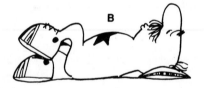

Body mechanics

The joints and bones in your body are parts of a machine that will wear out if they are strained too much or incorrectly. Also, advancing age and long-term use of steroids may make bones brittle. Proper body mechanics are essential to make the whole of your body function effectively.

It is important that your motions be smooth and steady, never jerky or sudden. Do not lift, push, or pull when your back is twisted or bent. Use your feet to turn around, and lift by bending and straightening your knees. When you lift an object, it should be held as close to your body as possible.

Yes No

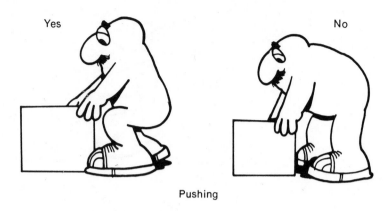

Pushing

Avoid carrying heavy items in your arms; instead, utilize a rolling cart of some kind for them (for example, for groceries, laundry, and equipment).

Yes No No

Working surfaces should be of the proper height so you can avoid excessive back bending or having to lift your arms too high. Proper working-area height is generally a couple of inches below your elbows, for both the standing and sitting positions.

Never sit in a chair that's too low; your back, feet, and arms should always be well supported. You will generally feel more comfortable sitting erect or even leaning slightly forward.

Redevelopment of Good Posture

Maintaining a well-balanced carriage is as essential to habitual good breathing as using your diaphragm and abdominal muscles and relaxing the shoulders, neck, and upper chest. The following basic points should be considered and practiced.

1. Stand with at least half the body weight carried forward over the forepart of the feet so that the toes are well pressed onto the ground.
2. Practice rocking forward until the heels have to come off the ground and backward until the toes do, then settle between these two extremes. The weight should be at least evenly divided between the front of the foot and the heel. In most cases it is necessary to accentuate the forward shifting of your weight.
3. Stand sideways in front of a long mirror and note:
    a. Is your head poking forward? Correct this by stretching upward and tucking your chin in while pressing your head backward.
    b. Is your seat sticking out? Tuck in the seat muscles and relax your shoulders and upper chest.
    c. Do your shoulders hunch forward? Bring your shoulder blades down and back.
4. When sitting in a chair, sit well back in the seat and support your legs on the floor (never dangle). Support your arms on armrests or place them on your lap.

Practice posture work against a wall for about 5 minutes at a time. Assume the following position.

1. Place feet a few inches apart and a few inches away from the wall.
2. Hold head high.
3. Tuck chin in.
4. Relax shoulders.
5. Tuck hips under.
6. Slightly flex knees.

When you feel you can hold the position properly, try standing away from the wall in the proper postural position, and then attempt to walk in this position. You will notice that the trunk stays quite rigid but the legs, both hips and knees, bend more when walking in this way. Check to see if you have retained the proper position by backing up to the wall frequently during your walking practice. Do not stiffen up when trying to maintain a proper posture. Only by being relaxed can you benefit from this exercise.

12

You Are What You Eat

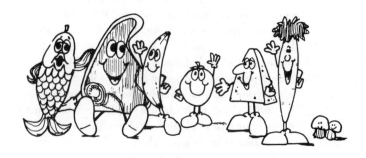

Eating good food is one of the great pleasures in life. What you eat affects the way you feel, your ability to fight infections and diseases, your emotional health, and, ultimately, the length of your life.

We are continually flooded with information about nutrition. Newspapers, magazines, radio, and television have advertisements, articles, and commentaries about the subject. Some of the information comes from reliable sources; a lot of it does not. Nutrition is now "in." It is big business. Whenever any health issue is popular, the public must be wary. People have to know who is saying what—and why. Daily, there are stories that say "don't eat this (it may kill you)" or "do eat that (it will cure whatever is wrong with you)." A person who reacts to all these stories can become confused at best and extremely anxious at worst. Unfortunately, most such information is incomplete or is based on either no scientific studies or a misinterpretation of the studies done. There is no question that good nutrition is important. There is also no question that there are well-meaning people who are convinced that eating sugar is "bad" or that taking large quantities of certain vitamins is "good." However, conviction, enthusiasm, and testimonials are no guarantee of scientific accuracy.

When it comes to a sensible approach to nutrition, a few facts about how the body works should be kept in mind. The first is that the body and its digestive system are very smart. Most of the things you eat can be converted from one form to another by the body. It is very difficult to trick the digestive system. For example, the body requires sugar as an energy source. If you take none in, the body will make it out of other things you eat—otherwise your "engine" would not run. Indeed, this ability of the digestive system to make the things it needs often saves us from ourselves when we go on strange fad diets. Given this marvelous, flexible manufacturing system, all we have to do to maintain good nutrition is to use common sense. Give the body an even break and it will serve you well. Therefore the basic rule of good nutrition is a simple one: *eat everything in moderation.* Fad diets and fear about eating certain things are not warranted. Unless you have some kind of rare digestive disease, are truly allergic to some food (a very rare situation), have some kind of hereditary problem (again, quite rare), or have special medical problems, eating a regular, reasonably balanced diet is all you need to do. *Just avoid excesses.* Eating a gallon of ice cream a day does not make sense, nor does being terrified of eating a dish of ice cream. Salting foods until they are white is not moderation. There is no reason to challenge your body. Treat it reasonably. Eat things in moderation.

It certainly is a fact that with decreased physical activity, you need fewer calories to burn for energy; yet you still need protein, carbohydrate, fats, vitamins, and minerals. You can manage this balancing act by avoiding an excess of foods that provide mainly calories but few nutrients, such as sweets, fast foods, and packaged "goodies." Give some thought to your choices and select those foods that give you more of the nutrients you need.

A very important goal for an individual with COPD is to maintain an ideal body weight. Being overweight causes the "engine" to work harder and makes the "work of breathing" more difficult. Being underweight robs you of the strength and endurance needed to combat fatigue and infection.

So, pay attention to the scale! Discuss your dietary goals with your physician. Perhaps he or she can suggest a nutritionist to help you reach your ideal body weight and to provide information about appropriate dietary habits.

The Six Essential Nutrients

There are six nutrients essential to health and life itself.

1. *Water* accounts for more than two thirds of your total weight. It not only helps to digest food and eliminate waste, but, for individuals with lung disease, it also helps to keep mucus and secretions thin. Without the thinning effect of liquids, mucus becomes thick and is a prime breeding ground for infection. What you drink is up to you and your individual needs. If you need to gain weight, milkshakes and nectars are appropriate. If you need to lose weight, stick to water and other low-calorie drinks. Remember that fluid is especially important for the individual with COPD.

2. *Protein* provides the eight essential amino acids your body needs for repairing its tissues. Milk and milk products, eggs, meat, fish and poultry contain all eight essential amino acids and are termed *complete*. Whole-grain breads and cereals, nuts, legumes, and dried beans provide useful but less-complete proteins. When combined in a meal these incomplete proteins become complete (with all the essential amino acids) and are fully utilized by the body. Whatever your protein choice, it's wise to make it a low-fat one. Choose meats that are less marbled. Remember to trim off all visible fat before cooking because this also trims fat calories.

3. *Carbohydrates* are the least expensive and most easily digested form of energy. All tissues require glucose (a simple carbohydrate) as a source of energy. Complex carbohydrates such as whole-grain breads and cereals, pastas, potatoes, rice, and fruit provide good-quality carbohydrates, as well as other nutrients. The soluble fiber in oats and brown rice may help lower your cholesterol level, which can reduce your risk of developing heart disease. The indigestible fiber in wheat bran helps with bowel elimination and may help protect you from certain cancers. Besides fiber, these foods are rich in vitamins and minerals and are good nutritional choices.

4. *Fats* are primarily a source of energy. They also contain, in their natural state, the essential fatty acids and act as carriers for the fat-soluble vitamins (A, D, E, and K). These vitamins are found in butter, margarine, meat, and vegetable oils. The "good" fats are monounsaturates—such as olive oil, canola oil, and peanut oil—and polyunsaturates—such as safflower oil. They also help to lower your blood cholesterol level. Saturated (hard) fats are the least desirable. Lard and hard fats (such as regular margarine, butter, and tropical oils) should be used sparingly if at all. Remember, it's saturated fat in the diet that leads to a high cholesterol level in the blood.

5. *Minerals* help build blood, bone, and teeth and aid in vital body functions. Calcium is a mineral that is often neglected by adults. Even though your bones are no longer growing, your body needs calcium because calcium can be withdrawn from the bones if your food does not provide enough to meet your needs. Calcium is also needed for normal blood clotting and for healthy nerve and muscle action. Drinking two 8-ounce glasses of milk or eating 3 ounces of cheese every day usually provides enough calcium.

However, some medications can interfere with calcium absorption, so be sure to discuss this with your physician. You don't need to worry about milk causing excessive mucus production—there is no scientific evidence to show that it does!

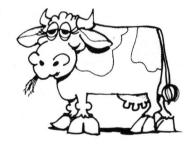

Iron is a mineral that is required for healthy blood and is often neglected in our diets. Liver is the best source of iron, but iron is also available in eggs, other meats, fish, whole grains, poultry, and dried fruits such as raisins.

6. *Vitamins* are essential for proper utilization of food and for healthy functioning of the body. Practically everything that goes on within our bodies requires the action of one or more vitamins.

Vitamin A is necessary for normal growth and good vision and to fight infection. It is found in butter and dark, leafy, green and yellow vegetables.

The B vitamins are necessary for nerve function, digestion, good appetite, and healthy skin. Whole-grain breads and cereals, meat, poultry, fish, nuts, and dairy products are the best sources of the B vitamins.

The amount of vitamin C needed is controversial. The best sources of vitamin C are the citrus fruits (oranges and grapefruits), papaya, strawberries, broccoli, and turnip greens. Be sure to eat two or three servings of these foods every day.

The amount of vitamin E needed and its benefits are also controversial. If you are considering supplementing your diet, check with you doctor first. The best food source of vitamin E is wheat germ. Other good sources are vegetable oils, nuts, and legumes.

All the vitamins are important, and they are easy to obtain by eating a well-balanced diet that includes a variety of foods. Excessive vitamin-pill consumption can be not only harmful but expensive.

When making your food selections, keep in mind that you usually get more nutrition for your money from foods that have not been extensively processed or created in a factory. In other words, 5 pounds of oranges cost about as much as a box of cookies; a 10-pound bag of potatoes costs less than a box of instant, dehydrated, mashed potatoes; and a quart of milk costs much less than a six-pack of cola drink.

Eating right is important for anyone, but it is extremely important for individuals with COPD. Not only should you eat a well-balanced diet, but you must also follow special nutritional guidelines because of your disease. Some nutritional problems and ways to overcome them are listed in the following section.

Distension

Eating too much at one time or eating certain foods can cause your stomach to become "bloated" (distended), limiting motion of your diaphragm and making it harder for you to breathe.

SOLUTION

1. Eat six small meals a day instead of three big ones. This is a good idea for another reason. Digesting food takes energy, which requires oxygen, so eating small meals uses up less oxygen.
2. Avoid the gas-forming foods that cause you discomfort. Some people are bothered by the following foods:

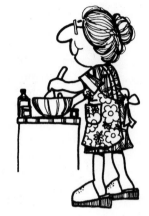

Brussels sprouts	Apples
Cabbage	Watermelon
Broccoli	Cantaloupe
Sauerkraut	Honeydew melon
Cauliflower	Some fruit juices
Asparagus	Onions
Beans	Radishes
Carbonated beverages	Beer
Excessive sweets	

3. Eat slowly and in a leisurely, relaxed atmosphere. If you rush through the meal or talk and chew at the same time, you might swallow air. Take time to enjoy your meals.
4. If the feeling of fullness continues from one meal to the next, you will need to eat food that leaves the stomach as quickly as possible. Fatty foods and fried foods should be avoided because they take longer to leave the stomach.
5. You can further reduce the volume of food in the stomach by taking liquids 1 hour before and 1 hour after, rather than during, the meal.

Loss of Muscle Mass

Because of the decreased activity of many patients with lung disease, their muscles become weak and flabby. Then, when they feel good enough to do something, they are too weak.

SOLUTION

1. Eat a well-balanced diet to obtain the proper vitamins and minerals.
2. Eat more high-protein foods such as meat, fish, poultry, and dairy products.
3. You can boost the protein and calorie content of your diet without greatly increasing the amount of food consumed. High-protein food additives, such as nonfat dried milk, may be added to sauces, gravies, creamed dishes, casseroles, puddings, custards, meatloaf, and other foods; you can add up to ¼ cup of the dried milk to many recipes without altering the favor.

4. Make "double-strength" milk by adding nonfat dried milk to regular milk, then mix well and chill.
5. Use milk, preferably "double-strength," instead of water for cooking cereals, diluting canned creamed soups, mixing puddings, and making instant cocoa.
6. Add small pieces of cooked meat to canned soups and casseroles.
7. Add grated cheese to vegetables, casseroles, and cream sauces.
8. Spread cream cheese or peanut butter on toast, whole-wheat bread, apple slices, fresh pears, or celery.
9. Use yogurt as a dressing for fruit salads. Cottage cheese and cream cheese make good combinations with fruit salads.
10. Add hard-cooked eggs to tuna and chicken, for either sandwiches or salads. Finely chopped egg may be added to sauces and some casseroles without altering the favor.

Loss of Appetite

Increased mucus production and some of the medications you take can result in appetite loss.

SOLUTION

1. Take medicines with milk or meals unless advised otherwise.
2. Exercise or practice bronchial drainage at least 1 hour before or after meals.
3. Drink a small glass of wine (not too much) before eating one meal.
4. Prepare foods with enticing aromas and vary your menus.
5. Food that is attractively served in a pleasant atmosphere is more tempting.
   a. Vary the colors and textures of food that is served.
   b. Use garnishes to brighten your plate.
   c. Colorful table settings, soft background music, and/or a change of location (a patio or sunny park) may make mealtime more enjoyable.
6. Get some fresh air and light exercise a short time before your meal.
7. Share a meal with a friend. Happy thoughts and pleasant feelings will help you enjoy your meal more and improve your appetite.
8. Take advantage of meals available at community centers, churches, and neighborhood schools. Call the American Lung Association, local health department, YMCA, or a local church for locations near you.

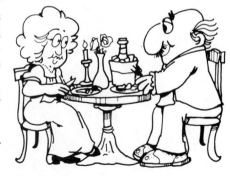

Hydration

Keeping secretions thin and easy to bring up is very important. If you do not drink enough fluids, your secretions will be thick and sticky and become a good breeding place for infections.

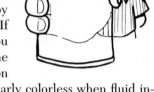

SOLUTION

1. Drink at least 1½ quarts of liquid each day. Besides water, you can drink fruit juices, nectars, milkshakes, and so on.
2. Check for dehydration (too little fluid) by watching for color changes in your urine. If your urine becomes a deeper yellow, you need to increase your intake of fluids. Urine color varies among individuals, depending on medication, vitamins, and so on; but it is nearly colorless when fluid intake is high.
3. When you have an infection or a fever, or when the weather is very hot, increase your fluid intake to 2 or 2½ quarts per day.

Potassium Depletion

If you use water pills (diuretics), you lose not only fluid but also potassium. When your potassium level is low, you might notice such symptoms as weakness, tingling, numbness of the fingers, or leg cramps. Low-potassium levels are also present in some individuals with COPD who are not taking medication.

SOLUTION

Eat several high-potassium foods every day.

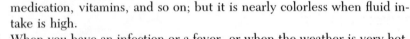

High-potassium Foods

Bananas	Peanuts	Beef
Oranges	Yams	Dried skim milk
Orange juice	Avocados	Winter squash
Raisins	Broccoli	Brussels sprouts
Dried apricots	Tomatoes	Pork
Dates	Potatoes	Chicken
Prunes	Fresh spinach	Fish
Cooked dried beans	Fresh mushrooms	Milk

Low-Salt Diet

Sometimes eating salt, even normal amounts, may cause you to retain excess fluid in your body. Your doctor will tell you if your condition, or certain medicines you take, may lead to this problem with salt. If the problem is not too great, just avoiding the salt shaker in cooking and at the table is often enough salt restriction. If your problem is more severe, you may need to avoid all salty foods (ham, luncheon meats, bacon, canned soups, snack foods, and convenience foods). Your doctor will tell you how much your salt intake should be restricted, and your dietitian will provide a specific low-salt diet to meet your needs.

Tips To Save Time and Energy

Meal preparation can be a real drain on your energy and leave you without the strength you need to enjoy your meal. The following solutions may be helpful:

1. One-dish meals (casseroles) are easy to prepare and clean up.
2. Prepare recipes in large quantities and freeze individual portions for reheating.
3. Make up your own "TV dinners" with leftover single servings, but don't rely on commercial TV dinners. Their nutritive value is less than what you prepare yourself, and many are very high in sodium.
4. Avoid the last-minute rush. Meal preparation is less tiring when some of the meal is partly or fully prepared in advance, such as the salad, dessert, or casserole.
5. Oven cooking is less tiring than stove-top cooking. You might also try a slow cooker or crock pot.

Supplemental Vitamins

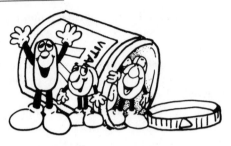

Large doses of vitamins and minerals are not recommended, but when food intake is limited, it might be necessary to take a daily vitamin and mineral supplement. It is particularly difficult to get the recommended amount of iron from the food you eat, so be sure your supplement includes it. Check with your doctor for his recommendations.

Good Luck!   **Good Health!**   **Good Eating!**

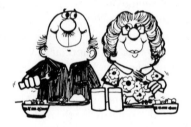

13

You Don't Have To Be Grounded

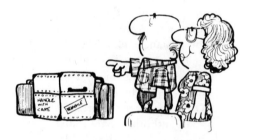

Travel is an important part of life for most people. You may need to travel for business purposes, to visit with family and friends, or just to enjoy "getting away" and seeing new places (or happy old ones). But when you have a breathing problem, the thought of leaving the security of home may prevent you from venturing out. Questions of safety, becoming ill, and needing help arise. For most people with COPD, however, there are relatively few contraindications to travel. With a little foresight and determination, you don't have to be grounded!

The most crucial consideration is that, while you can take a vacation, there is no vacation from respiratory care. You cannot tell your lungs that you are going on a trip and will return in 2 weeks. Although your daily routine will be interrupted, you must adhere as closely as possible to your respiratory-care routine. This means you must take your medications regularly and maintain hydration; if your routine includes bronchial drainage and breathing and physical training exercises, they must be continued.

The most important move you can make in planning a happy and healthy vacation is to consult your doctor, who will review your therapy and indicate whether any part of your program can be modified while you are away. Your doctor may want to give you the name of a physician at your destination whom you can contact if any difficulties arise, and he may even want to send a copy of your medical records ahead or with you.

In planning and preparing for your trip, you should consider some of the following travel tips:

TIP 1. When choosing your vacation site, check for the following:

Infections. Are there any viral flu epidemics at your destination? (Of course, you should check with your doctor about obtaining a yearly flu vaccine, regardless of known epidemics.) Does anyone you are going to visit have a cold? If so, you may want to postpone your trip.

Air pollution. How smoggy is the area? Will you have an air-conditioned room?

Allergy. If allergies play a part in your illness, avoid areas that have high-pollen counts.

Altitude. Consider the altitude of the area. As we ascend, air becomes less dense and there is less oxygen available to us. At short distances above sea level, this change is insignificant. But in cities at very high altitudes (that is, over 1-mile [5280 feet] high) or during air flight (cabins are pressurized to an atmosphere equal to about 1-mile high), the effect on people with COPD may be important, resulting in increased shortness of breath and other symptoms.

TIP 2. Discuss your trip with your doctor. Ask him for a written summary of your condition to carry with you. Ask how different altitude changes may affect you. If you need supplemental oxygen at higher altitudes, you must take it with you or arrange to have it there when you arrive.

TIP 3. If your doctor says that you need supplemental oxygen while flying, contact the airline *in advance*. Most airlines won't let you bring your own equipment on board. They will supply oxygen for you during the flight (but *not* during stop-overs or at your destination). They do charge for this service. Some airlines won't allow oxygen at all. Most require a written release from your doctor and information on the amount of oxygen to be used. A few even require accompaniment by a medical person or friend. *So check the rules well in advance.*

TIP 4. If you use oxygen or other respiratory equipment, ask your local vendor for the name of a company that will assist you at your destination. You may have to take some of your equipment with you, but you can arrange for whatever equipment and oxygen supplies you need to be waiting for you on your arrival. (Don't forget your cleaning supplies!)

TIP 5. Establish a travel routine for treatments, exercise, and cleaning of equipment. Write it down and follow it carefully.

TIP 6. Make a checklist of your medications. Take enough to last you for a few extra days in case of delay. It is occasionally difficult to get prescriptions from one state filled in another; nevertheless, obtain extra prescriptions from your doctor as another safeguard. Also, bring with you the over-the-counter medications you commonly use; for example, aspirin and antacids.

TIP 7. Travel is tiring; allow time for frequent rest stops. Relax and enjoy yourself. Don't try to do too much in one day; get adequate sleep.

TIP 8. Be prepared for climate and weather changes—for example, extra clothes for warmth.

TIP 9. Avoid smoking areas whenever possible, whether traveling by plane or train.

TIP 10. When traveling to foreign countries, avoid unknown medications, especially over-the-counter preparations that may contain substances that can cause harm. Be very sure to take a sufficient supply of all your medications if you are going to a foreign country.

• • •

Travel makes life interesting and rewarding. Travel whenever possible, but plan ahead.

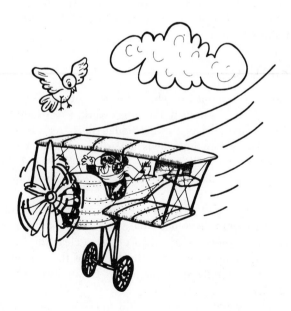

__ 14

Smoking, Smog, and Other Bad Stuff

One of the things you can do to help your lungs is to avoid certain things that may cause further irritation or damage. People with lung disease can't live in glass boxes, isolated from the rest of the world, nor should they try to. They shouldn't go around being afraid of every possible exposure. If you do that, your life will be full of fear and anger and no fun at all.

The causes of lung disease are complex. In fact, our understanding of what causes COPD and all the things that make it worse is far from complete. But we do know that certain inhalation exposures can make your lungs work less well. Sensible avoidance or prevention of these exposures can keep your lung problems from getting worse. But remember, becoming unduly fearful or angry can cause problems that are worse than the exposures themselves!

Smoking

Today, just about everybody knows that cigarettes can have multiple negative effects on the way the lungs work. For example, smoking can paralyze the hairlike cilia in the bronchial walls. As a result, these cilia cannot do their job of moving mucus toward the throat, where it can be eliminated easily. Mucus collects in the bronchial tubes and clogs up the bronchi, impairing movement of air and making the lungs more susceptible to infection.

Smoking also irritates the mucous-producing cells of the bronchi, stimulating them to produce excess mucus. This may further clog the lungs and lead to chronic cough, in an effort to clear the bronchi of mucus. In addition, smoking may cause the lining of the bronchial tubes to swell. This swelling (or inflammation) makes breathing more difficult and cough less effective.

People with COPD should not smoke. If you are still smoking, seek help in stopping. Call your local Lung Association, Heart Association, or Cancer Society. They may have classes or information available to help you. It is important *not* to feel angry at yourself or guilty or stupid for having smoked. Those kinds of negative feelings won't help you or your lung condition. Nor does it help to have other people, including your doctor, get angry at you and make you feel bad. Remember, most people have some habits they wish they could stop, too. No one is perfect. There is no question that you should stop smoking. Seek help in stopping. It's hard to do alone. Sooner or later you will succeed. But it's easier to succeed if you keep your self-esteem and are honest about the problem. There is no question that smoking makes your lungs function less well. You know that. So try, try, try. Those around you should work with you. Maybe you can help *them* overcome some of their bad habits the same way—with gentle, positive encouragement.

Cigarette smoking is not the only risk factor in chronic lung disease. Other factors, such as a deficiency of an enzyme in the blood, α-1-antitrypsin, can predispose a person to the development of emphysema. Smoking, however, is by far the most important risk factor.

Lung cancer is another problem linked to smoking. Cancer-causing elements, known as carcinogens, are found in cigarette smoke. These chemical agents may cause normal cells to develop into cancerous ones. Statistically, smokers have a far greater chance of developing cancer of the lungs than nonsmokers. Lung cancer has been a leading cause of death among American males for some years. The number of women with this disease has increased as they have taken up the smoking habit.

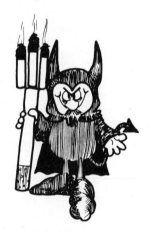

People with lung disease who continue to smoke are engaging in behavior that limits the benefit of treatments administered by their physicians.

The benefits derived from giving up the smoking habit are great. You may actually improve your lung condition! The risk of heart disease, cancer, and the development of further lung disease may be reduced. Coughing episodes and mucus production will decrease. Your ability to breathe will improve, thereby reducing the disability from your lung disease. It's worth it!

Environmental Exposure

Your breathing may be affected by a variety of factors found in the environment—for example, temperature and humidity. These factors may affect some people but not others; that is, the response to a certain environment is highly individual. Because we are all affected differently, it follows that there is no such thing as an ideal climate or environment for all COPD patients. The environment in which you feel most comfortable is the best for you. Let's look at some of the environmental factors that may influence your breathing.

Second-hand smoke

Unfortunately, you may be bothered by smoking even though you've given up the habit. This can happen when you are exposed to the smoke generated by others. Second-hand smoke may bother you psychologically in any concentration; high concentrations may make you feel more short of breath. If this is the case, you should steer clear of smoke-filled places. Also, don't be afraid to tell others that their smoking is bothering you. Telling friends, "Yes, I mind if you smoke!" is especially difficult at first. But with a little practice, you can manage. Here are some pointers. Be polite. Many smokers are not aware of the discomfort you may experience and will respect your request. Placing a "No Smoking" sign on your door or desk may be all that is necessary with friends. If you occasionally meet with a hostile response, remember that these people are probably not any nicer about this than they are about anything else. Seek out well-ventilated restaurants or "No Smoking" areas in restaurants and other public places. But avoid panic when exposed to smoke; that can be worse than any effect of smoke itself. Work yourself, and with others, to educate smokers about how you feel and why your desire for a nonsmoke environment should be honored.

Air pollution

Air pollution affects everyone, but research suggests that some people with asthma, chronic bronchitis, and emphysema may have more trouble breathing and increased coughing on days of heavy air pollution. The four major pollutants are sulfates, ozone, particulates, and carbon monoxide, primarily from factories and automobile exhaust. Carbon monoxide from car exhaust interferes with the blood's ability to carry oxygen. When this dirty air is exposed to the hot sun, it becomes even more irritating.

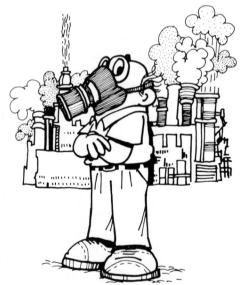

During "smog alerts" when air pollution rises to an unhealthy level, people with heart and lung disease are advised to stay indoors and avoid heavy exertion. Air conditioning in your home may help. It is also advisable to avoid rush-hour traffic, when automobile exhaust is worse. If you plan to travel, consider the air quality of the places you are visiting.

Industrial pollution

This occurs when the air in your place of work bothers your breathing. Your breathing may be affected by dusts, fumes, and gases and vapors from chemicals. There are some well-known kinds of industrial pollution such as exposure to asbestos or coal dust; but often the exposure is unreported. New forms are discovered every day. Therefore, if the air in your work place bothers you, you need to do something about it. See what dust and fumes might be produced in your work place. If possible, have them eliminated—at least, have ventilation improved. It may take some detective work, but it needs to be done.

Temperature

Some people are affected by temperature. Very cold air has been known to cause bronchospasm. Temperatures over 90° F can also affect your breathing and cause dehydration.

Wet vs. dry climates

The only person who can tell if a wet or dry climate is better for your breathing is *you*. You should visit both climates and decide.

Allergy

True allergies are abnormal responses to materials that exist in the environment. For example, onions make everyone's eyes water; that is not an allergy but an *irritation*. It is sometimes difficult to distinguish between irritation and true allergy. If you sneeze, develop a runny nose, have itching eyes or wheezing on exposure to things *that cause no symptoms in others* (for example, flowers, cats, or certain foods), you may have an allergy. Obviously, the best thing to do about allergies is to *avoid them* when possible. When avoidance isn't possible, allergies can be controlled with medicines such as antihistamines and corticosteroids. Most people with COPD (usually asthmatics) know what their allergies are and live with them.

It would be nice if we could escape to an environment that was ideal for everyone. But because we can't, we must each learn to make the one we have as healthy as possible.

Infections

Infections of the lungs can be caused by viruses, fungi, or bacteria. People with lung disease often have more severe symptoms with infection because their lung function is already decreased. Therefore it is important to report symptoms of infection promptly so that the cause can be identified and proper treatment started.

Viruses cause colds that may involve not only the nasal passages but also the lungs. There are no vaccinations or "shots" that prevent *all* colds. There is a vaccine that can prevent colds resulting from some kinds of influenza viruses. Every year a new influenza vaccine is made. It provides protection against those kinds of influenza viruses expected to occur that particular winter season. Most patients with lung disease should receive a "flu shot" each fall—unless they have problems with vaccines.

There is no pneumonia vaccine. However, one vaccine does provide protection against one kind of pneumonia, caused by bacteria called *pneumococci.*

Antibiotics are effective against bacteria and some fungi but not viruses. (Drugs that affect some viruses are also now available.) But because bacterial infections may follow virus infections, patients with lung disease sometimes are given antibiotics when they have colds.

You should talk with your doctor about when—and whether—you should receive these vaccines or antibiotics.

15

The Psychology of Better Breathing

If a man does not keep pace with his companions, perhaps it is because he hears a different drummer.

H.D. Thoreau

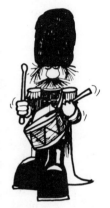

All of us would like to be able to do *what* we want, *when* we want, and *how* we want to do it. Unfortunately, we learn that many factors impose limitations. How we deal with these limitations determines how happy, productive, and pleasant our lives are.

Our state of health is one factor that can impose a significant limitation, and any chronic illness, such as COPD, imposes those limits permanently. A chronic limitation can be particularly difficult to deal with and can make individuals angry, anxious, and depressed. Although this is understandable, it is unfortunate, because the mind and body are closely interrelated. That is, physical health can influence mental health—and vice versa. This is particularly true for patients with COPD. Emotions can influence breathing in people with *normal* lungs, but they can have *major* effects on breathing when COPD is present. Therefore dealing with your emotional or psychological self is very important to your physical health.

Saying "Deal with your emotions" or "Learn how to live with limitations" is easy; *doing* it is difficult. This chapter may help you to do so by explaining the emotional problems common to persons with COPD.

In the main, you may face two kinds of problems: how you view yourself and how you relate to others.

You—The Person with COPD

We all have a certain image of ourselves physically and emotionally. That image is critical to how we function and how we relate to others, because our self-esteem is based on it. COPD may be associated with a number of changes in physical image. You may gain weight because of inactivity or steroid medications, or you may lose weight because of decreased appetite.

93

You may have noisy breathing, or you may cough and produce sputum. You may have to walk and do other things more slowly. You may need to use oxygen in public. All of these things may impair your physical image and cause you to feel unattractive and odd. If you feel this way, you may think that others see you the same way, and your self-esteem will suffer. *The first thing to recognize is that other people have a lot to think about besides how you look and breathe.* If they do notice and ask questions, such curiosity on their part is normal. It can be satisfied by telling them the truth. You can calmly say, "It's all right, I have a lung condition and need to use oxygen"; or "It makes me cough more than I would like." Most people understand and will easily accept the truth—and you. The people who count will accept individuals for what they are, not how they look. People who wear casts on their legs are always asked "What happened?" A straight answer ends the curiosity and normal interpersonal relationships resume.

Another limitation that can bother people with COPD is their vulnerability to things over which they have no direct control. All of us are vulnerable to a number of outside forces. But with COPD, many factors may pose a special threat to well-being: for example, infectious agents, atmospheric conditions, and environmental pollutants. Such factors may lead to unpredictable changes in daily activities, which are irritating if you are used to being organized and to carefully planning your daily activities.

COPD may lead to other alterations that can impair self-esteem. You may need to modify your work schedule or seek early retirement. You may need to modify or eliminate certain pleasurable activities: tennis, golfing, bowling, climbing, and other forms of recreation. You may need to explore a change in location to seek a more favorable climate, causing you to leave behind friends and familiar surroundings. These changes can cause periods of depression, which practically all people with COPD experience.

Depression involves feelings of sadness, hopelessness, and worthlessness. The symptoms are subtle in the beginning, consisting of a lack of interest in things (including your personal appearance, food, and outside activities) and fatigue. Going out becomes a chore; friends and hobbies are dropped. Everything becomes too much effort. Depression needs to be recognized early. Unless it is, inactivity results, which can worsen your condition. There is no easy antidote. You must force yourself to start moving, call friends, and go out; and, if necessary, seek outside counseling.

Certain phobias (abnormal fears of common experiences) may develop because of the real fear of becoming short of breath. For example, panic may be associated with entering closed spaces, even a shower stall. This panic worsens shortness of breath, and a terrifyingly vicious cycle of fear and further difficulty in breathing can result. This cycle can be prevented by learning how to control such situations with proper relaxation and breathing techniques.

Another common response to COPD (or any chronic illness) is denial. It is certainly useful to avoid becoming totally preoccupied with yourself and your illness. But denying illness can be hazardous if it leads to forgetting medicines, treatments, doctor's appointments, and real limits on your activity. It may lead to hiding your limitations from other people. You need to strike a balance between living with your limitations and denying their existence.

How You Relate to Others: The Spouse

Pulmonary illness has an impact not only on you but also on the others in your immediate family because it often alters the roles you play in relationship to others. For example, in marriage each partner usually accepts certain responsibilities. Each partner comes to rely on the other for certain activities. One may deal with finances and with social arrangements, whereas the other may deal more effectively with certain problems, people, house maintenance, or shopping. When pulmonary illness occurs, the nature of this sharing may need to change, temporarily or permanently. The spouse may have to assume new roles. There is danger in this situation for both patient and spouse. The patient may become more and more dependent on the healthier spouse (who, in turn, may become essentially a full-time nurse). The one with COPD may fear being left alone and require more and more from the spouse, including giving up his or her outside activities and work. Both resent the situation (often quietly)—one is angry about being dependent, the other is angry about becoming so depended upon. The answer is to discuss what is going on in the marriage. Excessive dependence (or doting) is to be discouraged. Both partners should do their share, even if those shares are modified in amount or nature.

Sex

To maintain an active, enjoyable sexual life there are also certain changes that a couple may have to make when one member has pulmonary illness. They may not be able to perform some of their previous sexual practices because the extent of exercise tolerance may be diminished. The length of time spent in activities such as foreplay may have to be modified. In addition, certain positions used during intercourse may no longer be comfortable and a change may be necessary. But there is no way that modifications can be made in sexual activity unless the couple is open enough to talk about sex. An unfortunate type of communication that couples frequently engage in is a game called "I hope you can read my mind." That is, one partner wants something changed sexually and hopes that the spouse will comply with the unspoken wish. The ice may have to be broken by one person just coming out and talking about it. For example, one woman was required to use oxygen for any type of exertion, including sexual activity. She felt that having her oxygen tank in the bedroom detracted from the sexual atmosphere during relations with her husband. Her solution was to place the tank outside the bedroom and use a long tube that reached the bed. There is no reason for sexual activity to stop because a person has pulmonary illness. The key is to be open about it, and modify the activity to that which is physically possible.

Friends

If you have a negative image of yourself, it may interfere with your friendships. You may begin to fear that you are more trouble than you are worth, that you are a burden to others. Your response may be to withdraw from relationships or to try to maintain a facade (doing more than you should really do). Again, the fact is that your friends rarely share your feelings (that you are a burden) and will respect and understand your limits. If you ask them to walk slower, to not smoke around you, or to alter social plans, almost all will understand and respond. But you can't play "read my mind." You must tell them of your limits, not hide them. You can take an active role in planning your social life so that it fits within your limitations. There is no need to be totally left out.

The Bottom Line

We have reviewed some of the common problems faced by patients with pulmonary illness and some of the feelings they may develop. There are some very important principles to remember to help you maintain both a positive state of mental health and a positive quality of life. First, having a pulmonary illness does not necessarily mean you must give up certain activities in your life. Instead you should *modify* the activity and *still be involved in it*. Many people have difficulty learning to pace themselves, but with patience and practice, it can be done. For example, people who are distraught that they can no longer play 18 holes of golf find that it is possible to play 9 holes with a cart. Patient and spouse can enjoy golf again, a pleasure they thought was gone forever. When you have pulmonary illness, you may develop misconceptions as to the safe limits of physical exertion; that is, once you begin to develop shortness of breath, you may stop the activity instead of slowing it down. There is a tendency to stop sooner and sooner during the activity, and consequently, to begin to feel that you can do very little. Although you may have to slow down, you can learn that, if you push yourself a little, you can do more than you thought. Doing more will improve your self-esteem and endurance. The important thing is to figure out *how* you can do what you like. Don't give it up! Rearrange it! Adapt it to you! Soon the pace will no longer be planned; it will become natural to you. You can continue to be involved with the world, with your family, and with your friends.

Another important principle is to learn as much as possible about your illness. You should try to learn about your lung function, your medicines, and your treatments. Ask questions of doctors, nurses, therapists, and other people with COPD until answers have been obtained. The process of education concerning your illness has an enormous psychological value. As you know more about your illness, some unfounded fears can be dispelled. In addition, as you develop more understanding, you can play a more active role in keeping yourself healthy and helping yourself when you are ill. A great deal can be learned not only from medical personnel, but from other patients as well. People with COPD have accumulated a vast amount of experience about how to live successfully within the physical 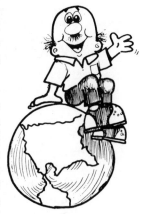 limits that exist. You can share their experiences, contribute your own, and give each other support. This can be done through rehabilitation programs, American Lung Association meetings, and informal groups.

The essence of good psychological health is to maintain a positive attitude toward living, while knowing the facts and being realistic. Remain as active as possible, and try to maintain your sense of humor. Your life is not "over" with pulmonary illness—it is *changed*, but you can enjoy this changed life greatly if you maintain a positive image of yourself.

16

When To Call Your Doctor and What To Do In An Emergency

Most people with COPD have regularly scheduled visits with their doctors. But when should you call him between these visits? Usually, in discussions with your doctor, signals are worked out to cover this question. In general, however, there are two major signals that your doctor will want to know about: (1) any *change* in your symptoms, particularly if this change lasts more than 1 day and (2) any *new* symptoms that you develop. Obviously, we all have our ups and downs, our good and bad days. But changes and new symptoms should be called to your doctor's attention.

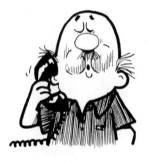

Some of the *changes* or *new symptoms* that might be important are:

Fever

Increased shortness of breath, difficulty in breathing, wheezing (more than usual)

Increased coughing (more frequent, more severe, or both)

Increased sputum production

Change in color of sputum (to yellow, gray, or green)

Change in consistency of sputum (thicker)

Swelling of ankles or legs or around eyes

Sudden weight gain (3 to 5 pounds overnight)

Palpitations of the heart or faster pulse than usual

Unusual dizziness, sleepiness, headaches, visual disturbances, irritability, or trouble thinking

Loss of appetite (more than usual)

Dehydration evidence by concentrated urine and dryness of skin

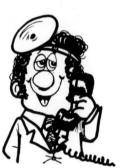

Chest pains

Blood in sputum, urine, or bowel movement

You should discuss these signals with your doctor, who may want you to change your medicines or add new ones (for example, to increase fluid intake and/or to start a preselected antibiotic for fever and increased cough). The more you work out these signals ahead of time, the better you will be able to deal with these changes, and the less frequently you will have to call your doctor on an emergency basis. **But when in doubt, check it out with your doctor.**

What To Do in an Emergency

Many patients and their spouses and family members want to know what to do in an emergency. There are two things that will make it rather simple to deal with this question: (1) become familiar with what an emergency is and (2) know what options for medical care are open to you and have a *plan.*

In general, an emergency is some *sudden* change or *new* development in your condition, particularly changes or new things that impair your ability to function or that frighten you. Sudden and/or severe chest pains or shortness of breath are the most common emergencies in COPD patients. Coughing up blood is another. *Sudden* changes in your condition and *new symptoms* of a major kind usually constitute a true emergency.

Of course, many patients with lung disease have mild changes that are frightening and may cause panic. Other sections of this book offer methods for dealing with panic. For example, if breathing becomes more difficult, you should assume a sitting position and lean forward slightly; pursed lip breathing usually helps, as may relaxation techniques (see Chapter 10). Inhalation of a bronchodilator aerosol (see Chapter 5) is useful if the shortness of breath is caused by bronchospasm. You must learn how to deal with such episodes; discussions with your doctor about these and other maneuvers will help.

But what if the symptoms are severe, don't go away, or are new? This constitutes a true emergency. In this situation, most patients want to see their doctor *immediately,* and that is a good idea because he or she knows you best. But that may be impossible or not in your best interests in an emergency. The key to constructing an emergency plan is, again, a discussion with your doctor. You should determine: when he is available (no one is available 24 hours a day, 7 days a week!); how you can contact him; and, if he is not available when you try to contact him, what you should do. Many doctors have associates who take calls when they themselves are not available; some do not. If you cannot contact him (or his associates), what should you do—call an ambulance or the paramedics? If you do that, to what emergency facility should you be taken?

The answer to these questions will be different in different communi-

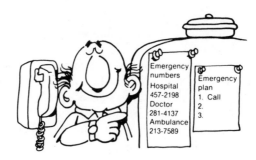

ties. In general, an emergency means you need prompt access to medical care. Obviously, it is an advantage if your doctor (or his associates) is available to provide your medical history, even if he cannot be physically present.

Therefore the important thing is to *plan ahead* so that you know what to do. Have a written plan near the telephone—names of *whom* to call and the proper telephone numbers: your primary doctor, backup doctors, ambulance or paramedic numbers, and location of the nearest emergency facility. Think through the situation ahead of time; put yourself in the place of your spouse or friend, as if you were helping *them* in an emergency. Once you have a plan, there is no reason for anyone to panic in an emergency. So worry about it *now* and get it worked out *now*. Hopefully, you will never need to put it into action!

Many patients don't want to "bother" their doctor; but whether your symptoms warrant "bothering" your doctor should be decided by the doctor. As you get to know each other and you become more knowledgeable, this decision will become easier. But err on the side of "bothering" whenever you are uncertain.

__ 17

Getting It All Together

Now that you have been introduced to the various methods of handling your COPD, you must learn to fit them into one day. Writing out a daily schedule is one method of helping you develop a *workable,* balanced regimen of treatments, rest, exercise, and recreation. Start by listing what you need to do each day. All the key elements of *your* particular program should be included, whether they consist of medications alone or include such things 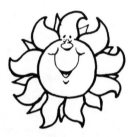 as bronchial drainage, breathing exercises, aerosol treatments, body improvement exercises, walks, special meals, and so on.

The schedule should be set up realistically so that you can follow it with as little frustration as possible. You should remember that you will have to push yourself at times and you *will* have to work—but the rewards will be plentiful!

The sequence of your program is important. Here are some tips to remember in setting up your daily schedule:

Bronchial drainage (as you have learned in Chapter 9) should never be done on a full stomach. It should be performed before meals or 1 hour after meals.

Medication (pills) to open your airways (bronchodilators) should be taken at least ½ hour before doing each bronchial drainage treatment. This will help to widen the airways and therefore drain the mucus more effectively.

Inhaled bronchodilators and mist-producing machines (for instance, nebulizers) should be scheduled for use before the bronchial drainage treatment and generally before exercise.

Never *exercise* or walk immediately after a meal. Wait for an hour or so; or do your exercises before the meal.

Remember to schedule *naps* and *rest* periods, as well as snacks and fluids, throughout the day!

An example of a typical daily schedule is shown on the following page.

With the help of your doctor, nurse, or therapist, fill out the blank schedule form, using the example as a guide.

Sample Schedule

MORNING

1. After awakening, take bronchodilator medication (pill), if prescribed.
2. Use inhaled bronchodilator, if prescribed.
3. Do bronchial drainage immediately afterward.
4. Breakfast.
5. After an hour or so, walk at designated speed and time. (Practice breathing exercises while walking.)
6. Have a nutritious snack with a glass of liquid.
7. Rest.
8. Liquids. (Space liquid intake throughout day and keep a careful record of amounts).
9. After you feel rested, perform body-improvement exercise(s).

AFTERNOON

1. Lunch.
2. Medications.
3. After an hour or so, practice breathing exercises and relaxation techniques in a quiet setting.
4. Walk at designated speed and time. (Remember breathing exercises while walking.)
5. Snack, with a glass of liquid.
6. Body improvement exercise(s).
7. Liquids.

EVENING

1. Dinner.
2. After an hour or so, walk again at designated speed and time.
3. Do arm exercises.
4. Medications.
5. An hour or more before bedtime, use bronchodilator aerosol.
6. Do bronchial drainage immediately afterward.
7. Perform body improvement exercises.
8. Clean nebulizer equipment (if applicable).

Modifying Your Schedule

If you're a working person you will have to adapt your daily program of care within certain constraints. For example:

1. Get up earlier to allow plenty of time to do bronchial drainage thoroughly. You'll feel more like "tackling" the day if your lungs are not full of mucus.
2. If bronchial drainage isn't a part of your program, get up earlier to take your walk before getting ready for work.
3. Arrange to take one shorter walk at lunch time, then eat your lunch afterward.
4. A good way to remind yourself to take liquid throughout the day is to have a pitcher or thermos of water, juice, or other beverages readily available on your desk or nearby.
5. At break time, find a quiet place where you can totally relax. Practice your relaxation techniques or your breathing exercises at this time.
6. Do your breathing techniques throughout the day while working.
7. After arriving home and relaxing a bit, take another walk right before dinner.

Don't forget time for *you!* Arrange your schedule so that it includes time for some of your favorite hobbies and activities. These are important for your mental health!

Your Daily Schedule

MORNING

1. _____
2. _____
3. _____
4. _____
5. _____
6. _____

AFTERNOON

1. _____
2. _____
3. _____
4. _____

5. _____

6. _____

EVENING

1. _____

2. _____

3. _____

4. _____

5. _____

6. _____

18

You Don't Have To Do It Alone—Pulmonary Rehabilitation

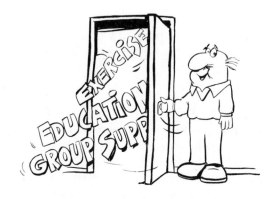

So far in this book we have discussed some general and specific health-care measures that are important for the person with COPD. Learning more about COPD and your own condition is an important step in improving your quality of life. In many areas, pulmonary rehabilitation programs run by health professionals who are experienced in helping patients with lung diseases have been established. Their goal is to help patients learn more about their disease and to cope better with it.

Rehabilitation is defined as "the restoration of the individual to the fullest medical, mental, emotional, social, and vocational potential of which he or she is capable." A *pulmonary* rehabilitation program is one which specializes in the rehabilitation of individuals with chronic lung disease.

People with COPD, like all individuals, can live fuller and more productive lives if they *actively* participate in their own health care and have the *tools* by which to do so. Pulmonary rehabilitation is a preventive health-care program provided by a team of health professionals, a program designed to help you acquire these tools. The primary goals of a pulmonary rehabilitation program are to provide you with the proper information, education, specific self-care therapies, and support to help stabilize your illness and improve your quality of life. Specific aims of pulmonary rehabilitation are as follows:

1. To teach patients, their family members, and significant others about COPD, its effects and consequences, and ways to minimize or control the problems that COPD may cause.
2. To maximize physical strength and tolerance for exercise.
3. To reduce symptoms and help you gain control over them.
4. To enhance emotional well-being.
5. To help you cope with the limitations and frustrations caused by having COPD.
6. To increase self-confidence and independence.
7. To help you become a more *active* partner in your relationship with your physician.

What are the Components of a Pulmonary Rehabilitation Program?

Evaluation

If you have COPD you can be considered for participation in a pulmonary rehabilitation program if you are *motivated* to learn more about your condition and to help yourself. An interview with a team member is an important part of the assessment process. During the interview, the program is explained, any questions are answered, and medical records are reviewed. A specific program can then be designed to meet *your* individual needs.

Physical therapy

Good bronchial hygiene, effective coughing, clapping, and bronchial drainage may be taught as part of a self-care program. Instruction in diaphragmatic breathing exercises and pursed lip breathing is stressed and reinforced. These measures are designed to reduce the work of breathing and to increase your ability to perform daily activities.

Respiratory therapy equipment

Instruction may be provided in the proper use and cleaning of respiratory therapy equipment (for example, metered dose inhaler, spacer, extender, or nebulizer). Your potential need for supplemental oxygen can be evaluated. If this or other equipment is needed, instruction will be provided regarding its proper use.

Education

Active patient participation is important. Therefore you and your family members should *understand* your underlying disease process, as well as the kinds of activity you can perform safely. Team members will discuss topics with you, such as the purpose of your medications and their side effects; proper nutrition; identifying signs and symptoms of a respiratory tract infection; and self-care tips. They will also help you to plan a daily schedule.

Exercise

A physical conditioning program is an important component of pulmonary rehabilitation because it has been shown to improve exercise capacity for individuals with COPD. After a thorough, initial evaluation, the team will select an appropriate and safe exercise routine tailored to your needs, supervise you during the initial stages, and prescribe a safe routine for you to follow at home.

Feelings and emotions

Successful rehabilitation requires attention not only to *physical* problems but also to *psychological, emotional,* and *social* ones. Understandably, individuals with chronic illness often have difficulty dealing with the limitations and symptoms caused by their illness. One symptom in particular, *shortness of breath,* is closely linked to your emotional state. The sensation of shortness of breath may lead to anxiety and fear, which may then cause more shortness of breath and discomfort—leading you to a vicious cycle. Support groups may help you to feel less isolated and alone. These groups also provide a forum in which you can share feelings, frustrations, hopes, and joys.

Benefits of Pulmonary Rehabilitation

Through the years, research has shown that there are measurable benefits from participating in a comprehensive pulmonary rehabilitation program. Some of these benefits are:

1. Increased knowledge about lung disease
2. Increased exercise capacity
3. Improved ability to perform activities of daily living
4. Decreased sensation of shortness of breath
5. Decreased anxiety and panic
6. Improved quality of life
7. Decreased time spent in hospitals

These benefits are certainly encouraging, but it must be stressed that it takes a motivated, commited person to participate in pulmonary rehabilitation and to make the necessary changes to improve his or her life. With a little help from a team of qualified, supportive, and caring health professionals, these benefits may be within your reach.

Where Are Pulmonary Rehabilitation Programs Located?

Pulmonary rehabilitation programs exist nationwide. Ask your physician, friends, local hospital, or American Lung Association for information on a nearby program. Also, the American Association of Cardiovascular and Pulmonary Rehabilitation publishes a nationwide directory.

If *you* are ready, there are programs ready for you!

19

A Look to the Future

Medical research is constantly working
toward the answers to many of the mys-
teries about COPD. Research on emphysema has indicated that the destruc-
tion of elastic tissue in the air sacs probably results from digestion of this tissue
by an enzyme called *elastase*. This enzyme is normally carried around the
body in white blood cells. We also know
that a blood protein called α-1-anti-
trypsin (also called α-1-proteinase inhib-

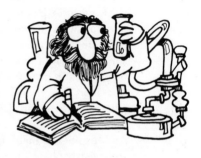

itor or "α-1-Pi") can inhibit (prevent or block) the effects of elastase. Some
persons have an inherited deficiency of α-1-Pi and experience emphysema
early in life, but this deficiency is rare. α-1-Pi has been purified and is now
available to give to individuals born with this deficiency. Why the elastase-
inhibitor system becomes unbalanced in patients who do not have a *hereditary* α-1-Pi deficiency is not clear. It is known that oxidants, including
those in cigarette smoke, can render α-1-Pi *inactive*. Intensive research is
focused on whether this inactivation, and other factors, lead to lung injury.
If we learn this, we should be able to develop drugs to prevent this injury.
Indeed, new drugs that block elastase and oxidants are under development.

The causes of chronic bronchitis also are being studied. Clearly, there
is an association with cigarette smoking and certain industrial exposures—
but why? What inhalants are responsible? What makes the bronchial tubes
behave the way they do? Can we develop drugs that will thin mucus effectively, prevent excess mucus production, or stop the inflammation of the
bronchial tube lining? We probably can and will.

Existing drugs and treatments for COPD are constantly being refined,
and new ones are being developed. Just within the last few years, several
new medicines have been introduced that relieve spasm of bronchial tubes
or relieve inflammation of the mucous membrane. These are better than
our older medicines in that they may have fewer side effects, may have a

longer duration of action, may be in a more convenient form to take, may prevent spasm (rather than treat it after it occurs), or may be more effective or less costly. Although "new" does not mean "better" by any means, some of these new medicines may be better for you.

Another example of what lies ahead concerns drugs for the improved treatment of infection. As discussed earlier, infections are caused by different kinds of invaders—bacteria, fungi, and viruses. Antibiotics are effective in treating infections caused by bacteria. Unfortunately, they are not that effective against fungi and are not useful at all against viruses. No antibiotic can treat the flu and other virus infections. But research already has provided some drugs that can prevent (or treat) certain kinds of virus and fungus infections, and the future in this area looks bright.

Lung transplantation is another area of intense interest. Questions that need answers include: Who *needs* a lung transplant? *When* should a transplant be performed? Is one "new" lung (vs. two) enough? How can we preserve a potential donor lung longer (currently, it must be used within 3 to 6 hours after removal)? How can we prevent lung rejection? Questions, questions, questions! All needing answers. In the meantime, a number of patients with severe COPD have received a lung transplant and the pace is accelerating.

Despite the many questions that remain, we clearly have made substantial gains. Some of the biggest gains are in the *education of the public* about the factors that contribute to the disease. Young children are being taught the hazards of smoking in the hope that they will never *begin* to smoke. Smokers are being aided in their efforts to quit. Many agencies are working toward cleaning up our air, another source of lung pollution.

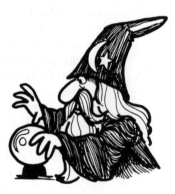

We are becoming aware of certain hazards to the lungs in the *workplace* (with asbestos being the most publicized) and are making progress in decreasing such hazards. Everywhere in our country, physicians and other medical personnel are becoming increasingly aware of COPD and are being trained in modern diagnosis and management techniques.

The more that medical research discovers about COPD, the better doctors will be able to treat their patients. The ultimate goal is to learn enough so that COPD can be prevented. The key to achieving that goal is to ensure that skilled researchers are trained and provided with the tools they need to continue the present pace of advancement.

Index